Information for Mental Health Providers Working with Children who have Chronic Illnesses

Author

Laura A. Nabors
Health Education Program
School of Human Services
University of Cincinnati
Cincinnati, Ohio
OH 45221-0068
USA

CONTENTS

CHAPTERS

Foreword by Keith A. King

Within this eBook, *"Information for Mental Health Providers Working with Children who have Chronic Illnesses"*, Dr. Laura A. Nabors reviews the critical role of mental health providers working with children who have chronic medical conditions in community settings, such as schools. A major focus is on presenting relevant, practice-oriented clinical research with case examples to illustrate key points in chapters. Dr. Nabors provides readers with an up-to-date review of issues and concerns commonly faced by children and families coping with a child's chronic medical condition. The ten chapters in this eBook effectively tackle a wide array of issues experienced by children, parents, and siblings. In carefully reviewing this eBook, I found it to be highly effective in displaying evidence-based content while also providing readers with practical strategies for effectively working with children with chronic medical conditions. In so doing, Dr. Nabors has greatly added to the professional literature by translating clinical research into professional practice. It is a hope that you will find this eBook to be as beneficial to your work as I have found it to be toward mine. There is no doubt that this eBook will benefit numerous health professionals, health educators, and mental health service providers.

Keith A. King
Professor and Program Director
Health Promotion and Education Program
University of Cincinnati
Cincinnati, Ohio
USA

Foreword by Jessica C. Kichler

In order to provide high quality mental health care for children with chronic medical conditions and their families, it is essential for mental health providers to stay up-to-date in their knowledge of clinical treatment practices and empirical outcomes. This eBook, entitled, *"Information for Mental Health Providers Working with Children who have Chronic Illnesses"*, summarizes the current literature related to helping children and their families cope with a chronic illness in multiple settings. Specifically, the eBook has a focus on the research outcomes associated with improving a child's adherence to medical regimens and his or her adjustment in the school setting. The eBook also addresses issues for the family members of a child with a chronic medical condition, including grief and parental and sibling adjustment. The purpose of the eBook is to provide information for mental health clinicians from a number of disciplines, including counseling and psychology. However, this knowledge is also useful for other providers on medical teams, who are assisting children in adjusting to and coping with having a chronic medical condition.

Ideas for improving child functioning are presented through case studies at the close of each chapter, which illuminates the most recent clinical perspectives in helping children cope with their chronic medical condition in real-world situations. A generalist perspective is used to illustrate multiple ways to help children with a wide variety of chronic medical conditions. However, there are also specific recommendations for helping children with different types of medical illnesses. Reintegration into their daily lives in ways to facilitate positive functioning and child resilience is an emphasis throughout several chapters. The eBook also provides vital resources on developing skills for a successful transition to adult care among children with chronic medical illnesses. Those who would like to learn even more about the different topics presented in the eBook can then consult the pertinent references presented within each chapter.

In summary, this eBook provides guidance to mental health clinicians working with children with chronic medical conditions in schools and private practice settings as well as those who work with children in hospital settings. The author's approach to this subject is both conceptual and practical and is aptly illustrated with case examples that are invaluable for clinical training. This eBook offers ideas for consideration for mental health clinicians of all experience levels and is a fundamental tool for those beginning in the field of providing specialty care to promote the mental health and functioning of children with chronic medical conditions.

Jessica C. Kichler
Pediatric Psychologist & Certified Diabetes Educator
Associate Professor of Pediatrics
Behavioral Medicine and Clinical Psychology
Cincinnati Children's Hospital Medical Center
Cincinnati, Ohio
USA

PREFACE

Children with medical problems often benefit from psycho-education and support from a mental health services provider. This eBook takes a broad perspective in reviewing roles for child mental health providers, such as a child psychologist or counselor who is working with children with medical problems. A non-categorical or generalist approach is a focus of chapters in this eBook, in order to broadly address ideas for mental health practitioners who wish to specialize in interventions for children who have chronic illnesses. Moreover, research examples and case studies also present information on the specific needs of each illness, which may be critical to helping children and their families. The author's goal is to provide a perspective that presents ideas for enhancing child functioning and mental health as well as encourage thought about the role of mental health providers in facilitation of the development of children with chronic illnesses as well as their families.

Suggestions for working with children and their parents, based on a review of relevant research are presented. An emphasis on supporting the child and enhancing resilience across key contexts for the child is provided. Improving communication between the medical team and school is another goal for improving child functioning. Assessment of child abilities and development of school care plans are steps in optimizing integration in school contexts. In addition, ideas for assisting children and families are presented through a review of case studies developed for teaching purposes (*i.e.*, these are not representative of actual client meetings or contacts). The importance of supporting the family, including siblings and parents, as well as the child with the illness, is emphasized.

Laura A. Nabors
Health Education Program
School of Human Services
University of Cincinnati
Cincinnati, Ohio
OH 45221-0068
USA

CHAPTER 1

Chronic Medical Problems and Their Impact on Children and Their Families

Laura A. Nabors[*]

Health Education Program, School of Human Services, University of Cincinnati, 468 Dyer Hall, Mail Location 0068, Cincinnati, Ohio, OH 45221-0068, USA

Abstract: This chapter reviews information about chronic medical problems and provides a definition of chronic illness. A philosophy of care, based on a systems approach for children with chronic illnesses is presented. Developing care plans aiming to integrate the child within his or her school and broader community are presented. Roles for mental health providers and ideas for promoting child resilience are outlined. Information in the chapters in this eBook is reviewed to orient the reader to upcoming material in this eBook.

Keywords: Children, chronic illness, mental health, promoting resilience, systems approach, teacher training.

INTRODUCTION

"About 10.3 million children and adolescents in the United States have chronic medical conditions, which involve issues with cognitive, physical, or social development (Algozzine & Ysseldyke, 2006)" [p. 217; Nabors *et al.*, 2008] A chronic medical condition has a biological cause, with physical symptoms that cause significant limitations in day to day functioning (Thies, 1999). "Children with chronic medical conditions suffer from symptoms that last for more than 3 months a year (Thompson & Gustafson, 1996) and these conditions include developmental illnesses (*e.g.*, cerebral palsy) and chronic diseases (*e.g.*, diabetes)" (Nabors *et al.*, 2008). When coping with school-related problems, children with chronic medical conditions can benefit from teacher assistance in improving their interpersonal functioning or academic performance and assistance when they

---

*Address correspondence to Laura A. Nabors:** Health Education Program, School of Human Services, University of Cincinnati, 468 Dyer Hall, Mail Location 0068, Cincinnati, Ohio, OH 45221-0068, USA; Tel: 513-556-5537; Fax: 513-556-3898; E-mail: naborsla@ucmail.uc.edu

must miss school due to medically-related absences (Power *et al.*, 2003). Furthermore, children who face illness cope with stress and are at an elevated risk for coping with psychological problems (Barlow & Ellard, 2006).

Children with chronic medical conditions are living longer and experiencing more opportunities to be integrated in school and in community-based activities (Thies, 1999)[1]. This allows for new challenges, such as maintaining peer relationships, keeping up with school work, and taking care of medical conditions in front of others. In terms of school absences, many children may miss class to attend doctor's visits or because they are hospitalized due to needing specialty care. In these situations, the family --- often the child, parents, and siblings --- must adjust to stressors and new environments (*e.g.*, hospitals and being away from home). This can be stressful and negatively impact coping of the child and others in the family.

The purpose of this eBook is to provide information for mental health professionals about psychological, social, and emotional issues faced by children with chronic medical conditions as they are integrated in their communities and schools. Additionally, a focus on resilience, for the child and family members, is evident in this eBook. Family resilience and positive coping enhances family functioning and thus other chapters focus on the impact of illness on parents and siblings. The transition to adulthood is an important one, and this is another key topic in this eBook. This eBook reviews ideas for health professionals interested in facilitating coping for children with medical problems. Much of the writing is influenced by research and information about care from the perspective of the pediatric psychologist or child health psychologist. The *Handbook of Pediatric Psychology, Fourth Edition*, edited by Michael Roberts and Ric Steele (2009) presents a good review of key topics in pediatric psychology and ideas for enhancing coping of children with different chronic medical conditions.

NON-CATEGORICAL APPROACH

In this eBook, a focus is a "non-categorical" approach, which is the idea that all children with chronic illnesses face some common stressors, such as worry about health outcome (Stein & Jessep, 1982). In contrast, an example of a specific,

---

[1]Material is reflected in a previous publication by Nabors *et al.*, (2008) in *Psychology in the Schools*.

illness-related stressor is concern about counting carbohydrates correctly for children coping with Type 1 Diabetes. Focusing solely on working with special issues related to Type 1 Diabetes is consistent with a categorical orientation toward working with children. A categorical approach considers each disease as being associated with specific problems, stressors, and medical challenges.

Material reviewed in chapters in this eBook address important topics for children with illnesses, with an emphasis on a non-categorical approach to steps for coping with chronic illness (Stein & Jessop, 1982). In Chapter **2**, social and developmental concerns for the child are reviewed. In Chapter **3** therapeutic interventions and ideas for assisting children with illnesses in coping with mental health problems are reviewed. Chapter **4** highlights ideas for care plans for children. Chapter **5** presents a review of literature emphasizing the importance of assessment of child functioning, including cognitive and achievement skills, at regular intervals. Chapter **6** discusses issues related to adhering to medical regimens and problems faced by the child's family. Chapter **7** expands on ideas related to family coping by addressing ways in which parents cope and adjust when their child has a chronic illness. Chapter **9** addresses an understudied area, transition to adult health care, which can be stressful for the child as services may not be as comprehensive as those provided during childhood. Finally, Chapter **10** presents a brief summary of the theory and key information presented in this eBook.

Although a non-categorical approach is beneficial in many ways and also great for general training purposes, there are times when a more categorical approach is appropriate. There are specific issues related to specific illnesses that children need to cope with. For example, children with Type 1 diabetes test their blood sugars in front of others, a unique issue. Children with cystic fibrosis often must eat a specific diet, which can be difficult to adhere to during the adolescent years. When specific issues are evident it is important for the mental health provider to be able to adopt a categorical approach, understanding the child's unique needs. Moreover, when a provider serves a specific team, he or she needs to endeavor to become an expert on the illness or illnesses the team is treating. Understanding medical aspects of treatment is important, in order to understand where the child and family are coming from and to do a good job of interacting with and sharing information about the illness with the medical team and others in the community.[1,2]

DEVELOPMENTAL SYSTEMS APPROACH

Bronfenbrenner's (1979) ecological model provides a theory to orient the therapist when he or she is working with children who have chronic medical conditions and their families. Anne Kazak and her colleagues have applied Bronfenbrenner's theory for pediatric specialists who work with children who have chronic medical conditions (Kazak *et al.*, 1995; Power *et al.*, 2003). "Adapting this model in a "chronic illness context" ensures that a clinician will remain family centered and consider the influence of multiple systems, including the school, neighborhood, and community on the child's interactions and development. In Bronfenbrenner's model, the child is at the center of several spheres of influence (*e.g.*, family, school). The child is nested within spheres of influence, including the family, hospital, school, neighborhood, and various social networks that influence a child's life." (source: Power *et al.*, 2003). Time is another key factor influencing how the child develops and reacts to spheres of influence in his or her life. For example, an eight-year-old may react differently to school absence and peer pressure than a fifteen-year-old based on his or her experiences and key figures in his or her life that influence adaptation. Fig. (**1**) presents this author's ideas of key spheres that influence a child. The circles represent some key spheres of influence in the child's (child represented as the star in Fig. **1**) life.

In Fig. (**1**), time is represented as a hashed line and it is the developmental changes a child undergoes as he or she ages. Thus, clinicians need to be aware that children experience chronic medical conditions differently, in terms of coping and the impact of the illness upon them, at different points or stages in their lives. Families, too, are at different points in their development when a child is diagnosed and faces certain challenges, and stage of family development may also influence child coping. This author also believes that many families and children with illnesses are characterized

---

[2]Material is represented in Bronfenbrenner (1979) in *The ecology of human development: Experiments by nature and design* and Power *et al.*, (2003) in *Promoting children's health: Integrating school, family, and community.*

by resilience. In Fig. (**1**), opportunities for resilience are represented by the crossed lines with arrows at each end.

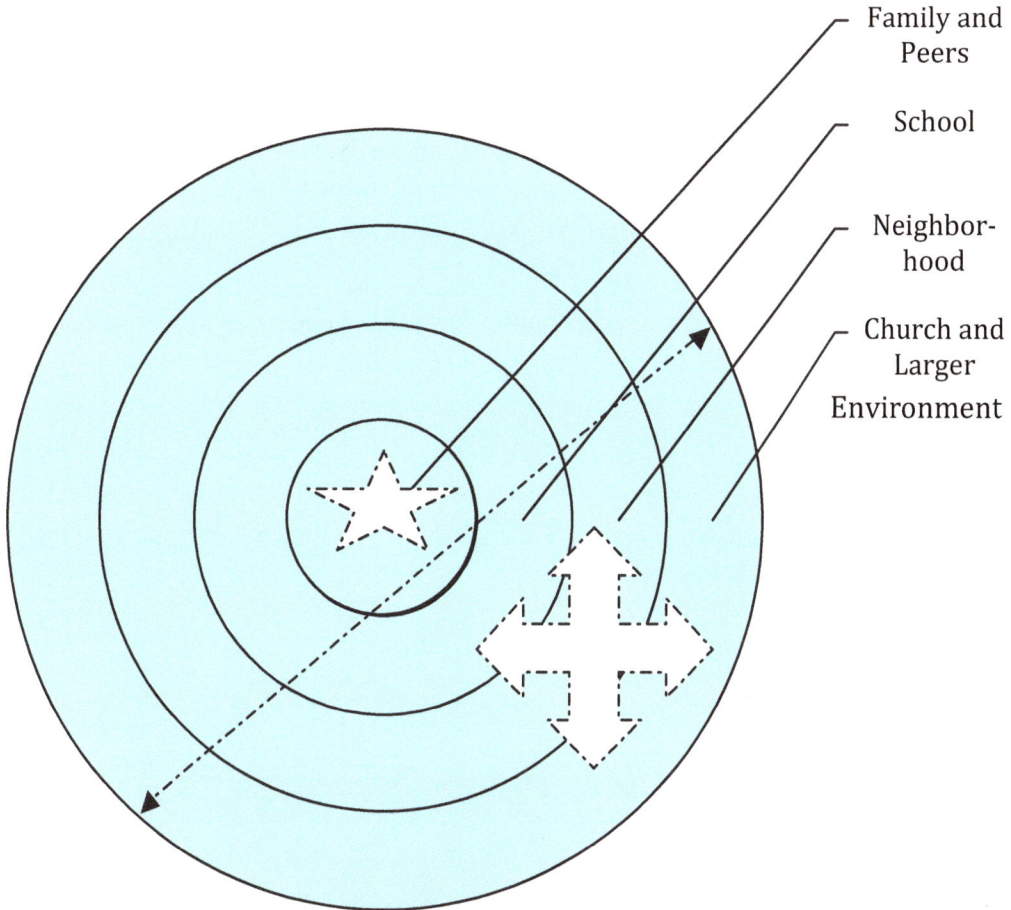

Figure 1: Critical Spheres of Influence for the Child. Note: The star represents the child, who is influenced by multiple spheres of influence in his or her environment.[1,2] The hashed line represents change over time as the child changes as he or she develops or ages. This figure represents this author's interpretation of "Bronfenbrenner's (1979) ground-breaking model." The crossed arrows represent how positive influences and experiences can increase resilience as the child interacts and changes through development.

Anne Masten has written extensively about resilience and describes resilience as a,

"…common phenomenon that results in most cases from the operation of basic human adaptational systems. If those systems are protected and in good working order, development is robust even in the face of severe adversity; if these major systems are impaired, antecedent or consequent to adversity, then the risk for developmental problems is much greater, particularly if the environmental hazards are prolonged" (p. 227).

Several factors can interact with resilient functioning. For instance, ethnicity can impact how resilience factors are perceived by children (Koninis-Mitchell *et al.*, 2012). Koninis-Mitchell *et al.*, (2012) also stated other child traits, including intellectual abilities or self-efficacy for disease management could be related to greater levels of resilience. Peer support may improve resilience; Fee and Hinton (2011) found that children who reported stronger peer support were functioning at a higher level. The aforementioned factors are intertwined with sphere or context influences that impact child adaptation and functioning. Resilience factors are building blocks of positive child functioning. As such, maximizing resilience factors and minimizing the impact of risk factors (*e.g.*, financial stressors) is one strategy for improving child functioning.

FAMILY UNIT AND SPHERES OF INFLUENCE

One might also conceptualize the family as a unit within a series of spheres of influence as illustrated in Fig. (**1**). If the family is also placed next to the child (represented as a star), then one can assume that the child and family unit are mutually influenced by the key contexts in their lives. This broadens the notion of spheres of influence as those spheres that influence parents, such as work, must also be considered. Considering family adaptation and resilience is critical, because the child and his or her family members reciprocally influence each other as they deal with the child's illness and other things that impact their lives (Rolland, 1984). To illustrate, the issues faced by a young family, with young children, are exacerbated by needing child care when the child with a chronic illness faces a medical emergency. In contrast, in a family where siblings are teenagers this is not an issue. Different issues, however, may emerge. Perhaps teenage siblings could feel shortchanged if parents could not chauffeur them to activities because they are attending to medical emergencies for their brother or sister who has a chronic illness.

Parent involvement in care of the child with a medical condition also differs based on child age and stage. Parents are primary caretakers when a child is young, but as the child becomes an adult, he or she becomes responsible for self-care. It may be difficult for some parents to adjust to this role change. Parent-child relations can be strained, if parents or caregivers and the young adult have different views about care of the medical condition. Thus, the notion that different reactions and coping skills are needed at different phases of illness adaptation is a key perspective for health professionals to consider when assisting a child and his or her family members adjust to a child's illness (Rolland, 1984). With the waxing and waning course of illnesses, phase of illness, individual and family differences to consider, addressing psychosocial issues for the child and family unit can be challenging. One possible approach is to "be there as needed, when needed". This type of "rubber band" approach allows the health provider to "pull tight" to help and provide education when needed, while allowing individuals and families opportunities to develop their own adjustment patterns as they adapt to the child's illness (see Nabors *et al.,* 2011).

INTEGRATION OF THE CHILD WITHIN THE COMMUNITY AND SCHOOL

Children with chronic illnesses may experience increased feelings of well-being and quality of life when they believe they are integrated with their peers in the community and school settings. Dr. Nabors has written extensively on the importance of integrating the child within his or her school and during community activities (*e.g.,* Nabors *et al.,* 2008; Nabors & Lehmkuhl, 2004). One way to facilitate this integration is to enhance communication between the child's primary, hospital-based medical team and providers (*e.g.,* teachers and school nurses) who are helping the child in community settings, such as school (Bradley-Klug *et al.,* 2013). Educating teachers and school nurses about the child's condition and care can also improve the medical care of the child at school. "Teachers are 'front-line' care providers and can benefit from knowledge about medical issues for the child and ideas for improving social integration of the child as well as the child's school performance (Clay *et al.,* 2004; Huffman *et al.,* 2003)" (source: Nabors *et al.,* 2008). Increasing school in-service training on health issues will improve school staff comfort and knowledge for assisting children with chronic illnesses as they navigate the complexities of managing school schedules, homework, after-school activities, and social support amidst the complexities of their chronic illnesses. The mental health provider also can intervene on a third level, working with the child and significant adults in his or her life to change a behavior. This can be done using reward charts, response prevention (*i.e.*, prevention of negative behaviors), as well as psychoeducational interventions.

Kazak *et al.*, (2010) recommended taking a "metasystems" approach when working with children and their families. Working with stakeholders and with making environmental changes in the many spheres of influence for the child and family (see Fig. 1) are helpful interventions and may at times be adjuncts to individual therapy. For example, if a child with juvenile idiopathic arthritis is having difficulty completing his or her homework, because textbooks are too heavy to carry home, then the professionals should work to assure that the child has an extra copy of books at home. Or, if the issue is that the child does not want to do his or her homework, regular communication between the teacher and parent may need to be established, perhaps through daily or weekly school to home notes describing the child's progress. The child is in a community, where he or she interacts in the neighborhood and participates in extracurricular activities – these settings may be areas for intervention to improve the inclusion of a child with a chronic illness. Thus, consideration of the adults and supports in each setting that is a key part of the child's life, and making adjustments or plans to improve child functioning across settings, is a key notion associated with taking a metasystems approach.

DEVELOPING CARE PLANS

In addition, "developing written care plans which outline the steps to illness management at school may provide extra support for the child [see Clay, 2004]" (source: Nabors *et al.*, 2008). A good example of key items to include in a written care plan for school are recommendations for routine care of the child's illness, daily medications, what to do in case of an emergency, whom to call in case of an emergency, and what to do when a child misses school in terms of helping the child complete missed assignments. The school nurse and each of the child's teachers should have a copy of the child's care plan. Care plans also should include a contact number for a representative of the child's medical team, in case questions arise. Care plans are essential components of a school plan that supports the child and informs others about how to assist the child. Care plans should be provided to coaches and after-school activity leaders should have a copy of the child's care plan and know how to help the child in case of a medical emergency.[1,2]

In order to inform parents in the neighborhood, or parents who may be caring for the child, the parent of the ill child needs to arrange an informal meeting or telephone conversation to explain his or her child's special needs. There should be ample opportunities for the other adults to ask questions and for discussion of whether the other adults are able to and are comfortable with assisting in management of the child's illness. If the other adults are not able to understand or commit to caring for the child, then meetings and play opportunities can occur at the home of the child who has special medical needs. However, efforts should be made to include the child in a normal routine, and help the child be integrated outside the home setting, so that inclusion occurs in as many settings as possible. The mental health professional can play a key role in assuring that key players in the child's life are linked to and in communication with the child's medical team. Improving understanding of the child's illness will ensure inclusion and increase the comfort and safety levels for the child and his or her family.

CONCLUSION

This initial chapter reviewed a "broad" definition of chronic illness and its impact on the child and family. A developmental systems approach to working with children with chronic illnesses is recommended, because it allows the clinician to help the child adjust to his or her age-related changes and consider the child's role within key systems in the community, such as school and after-school activities.[1,2] While the child is growing and changing, so are the family and parents and siblings. They undergo developmental changes as time marches on and they encounter different experiences in different settings. The role of a mental health clinician may be marked by flexibility. A rubber band approach may be advisable, with the clinician being there "as needed" to assist the child in coping with his or her illness at different developmental stages and under different conditions and to be there for the child's family as they undergo change and experience stress related to the child's chronic illness. Enhancing child resilience factors – to improve child coping and self-esteem –help the child thrive and can improve the child's efficacy for coping with his or her illness. Promoting inclusion of the child in community and school settings can enhance child well-being and psychosocial growth.

ACKNOWLEDGEMENTS

None declared.

CONFLICT OF INTEREST

The author confirms that this chapter contents have no conflict of interest.

REFERENCES

Algozzine, B., & Ysseldyke, J. (2006). *Teaching students with medical, physical, and multiple disabilities: A practical guide for every teacher.* Thousand Oaks, CA: Corwin.

Barlow, J. H., & Ellard, D. R. (2006). The psychosocial well-being of children with chronic disease, their parents and siblings: An overview of the research evidence base. *Child: Care, Health and Development, 32*, 19-31.

Bradley-Klug, K. L., Jeffries-DeLoatche, K. L., St. John Walsh, A., Bateman, L. P., Nadeau, J., Powers, D. J., & Cunningham, J. (2013). School psychologists' perceptions of primary care partnerships: Implications for building the collaborative bridge. *Special Issue in Advances in School Mental Health Promotion, entitled, Effectively Supporting youth with chronic illness in schools, 6*(1), 51-67.

Bronfenbrenner, U. (1979). *The ecology of human development: Experiments by nature and design.* New York: Harvard University Press.

Clay, D. L. (2004). *Helping schoolchildren with chronic health problems: A practical guide.* New York: Guilford.

Clay, D. L., Cortina, S., Harper, D. C., Cocco, K. M., & Drotar, D. (2004). Schoolteachers' experiences with childhood chronic illness. *Children's Health Care, 33*, 227-239.

Fee, R. J., & Hinton, V. J. (2011). Resilience in children diagnosed with a chronic neuromuscular disorder. *Journal of Developmental and Behavioral Pediatrics, 32*(9), 644-650.

Huffman, D. M., Fontaine, K. L., & Price, B. K. (2003). *Health problems in the classroom 6-12: An A-Z reference guide for educators.* Thousand Oaks, CA: Corwin.

Kazak, A. E., Segal-Andrews, A. M., & Johnson, K. (1995). Pediatric psychology research and practice: A family/systems approach. In M. C. Roberts (Ed.), *Handbook of pediatric psychology: Second edition* (pp. 84-104). New York: Guilford Press.

Kazak, A. E., Hoagwood, K., Weisz, J. R., Hood, K., Kratochwill, T. R., Vargas, L. A., & Banez, G. A. (2010). A meta-systems approach to evidence-based practice for children and adolescents. *American Psychologist, 65*(2), 85-97/ DOI:10.1037/a0017784.

Koinis-Mitchell, D., McQuaid, E. L., Jandasek, B., Kopel, S. J., Seifer, R., Klein, R. B., Potter, C., & Fritz, G. K. (2012). Identifying individual cultural and asthma-related risk and protective factors associated with resilient asthma outcomes in urban children and families. *Journal of Pediatric Psychology, 37*(4), 424-437. First published online March 9, 2012, *2012* DOI:10.1093/jpepsy/jss002.

Masten, A. S. (2001). Ordinary magic: Resilience processes in development. *American Psychologist, 56*(3), 227-238.

Nabors, L., Akin-Little, A., Little, S., & Iobst, E. (2008). Teachers' knowledge about chronic illnesses. For the mini-series: Psychology's contribution to education: Improving educational opportunities for all children. *Psychology in the Schools, 45*, 217-226.

Nabors, L., & Lehmkuhl, H. (2004). Children with chronic medical conditions: Recommendations for school mental health clinicians. *Journal of Developmental and Physical Disabilities, 16*, 1-15.

Nabors, L., Ritchey, P. N., Van Wassenhove, B., & Bartz, J. (2011). *Type I Diabetes in Children and Adolescents. In Chih-Pin Liu Editor. Type I Diabetes: Complications, pathogenesis, and alternative treatments.* (pp. 85-94). Croatia: In Tech.

Power, T. J., DuPaul, G. J., Shapiro, E. S., & Kazak, A. E. (2003). *Promoting children's health: Integrating school, family, and community.* New York: Guilford Press.

Roberts, M. C. & Steele, R. G. Eds. (2009). *Handbook of pediatric psychology: Fourth edition.* New York: Guilford Press.

Rolland, J. S. (1984). Toward a psychosocial typology of chronic life-threatening illness. *Family Systems Medicine, 2*(3), 245-262.

Stein, R. E., & Jessop, D. J. (1982). A non-categorical approach to chronic childhood illness. *Public Health Reports, 97*(4), 354-362.

Thies, K. M. (1999). Identifying the educational implications of chronic illness in school children. *Journal of School Health, 69*(10), 392-397.

Thompson, R. J., & Gustafson, K. E. (1996). *Adaptation to chronic childhood illness.* Washington, DC: American Psychological Association.

CHAPTER 2

Facilitating Child Coping with Chronic Illness

Laura A. Nabors[*]

Health Education Program, School of Human Services, University of Cincinnati, 468 Dyer Hall, Mail Location 0068, Cincinnati, Ohio, OH 45221-0068, USA

Abstract: Chapter **2** reviews research in key areas that are resilience factors for facilitating child coping with a chronic illness. For instance, positive social functioning is a component of successful adjustment that has a positive impact on developmental outcome. Enhancing the child's strengths and improving peer and family support are strategies for improving child functioning and resilience. Research on the effectiveness of support groups is presented and online support interventions are a method for reaching children who do not have access to support groups in their area. Helping children cope with grief and adjust to loss – associated with their chronic illness – is an area where mental health providers should develop skills, if they are interested in working with children who have chronic illnesses. Learning about interventions for improving emotional and behavioral functioning, especially coping with anxiety and depression in children, are other areas for skill-building.

Keywords: Child coping, chronic illness, emotional functioning, facilitating resilience, grief, peer support, social functioning, support groups.

INTRODUCTION

A child who has a chronic illness may face social and emotional challenges and the mental health provider can play a key role in helping the child toward positive adjustment and functioning amidst developmental change as well as illness-related crises. As mentioned in Chapter **1**, the mental health provider develops a "child and family support" orientation. When the child and his or her family are doing well the clinician's role is minimized; if this changes then the clinician can become more involved when either the child or family members experience developmental changes or issues related to the child's medical condition. Many

---

*Address correspondence to Laura A. Nabors: Health Education Program, School of Human Services, University of Cincinnati, 468 Dyer Hall, Mail Location 0068, Cincinnati, Ohio, OH 45221-0068, USA; Tel: 513-556-5537; Fax: 513-556-3898; E-mail: naborsla@ucmail.uc.edu

illnesses have a varied course, with waxing and waning of symptoms, and thus the mental health provider needs to assume a more supportive role when symptoms are strong and the child and family are experiencing stress related to worsening of the child's medical condition. Sudden shifts in the child's medical condition can take a toll on his or her social and emotional functioning. The mental health provider can provide the child with support to cope with the changing course of his or her illness. The mental health provider also can provide support to the child to improve his or her social and emotional functioning when the child is experiencing problems in either area.

SOCIAL FUNCTIONING

Many children who have a chronic illness do well socially; however, others can experience difficulties interacting with peers and being accepted by peers. Sentenac *et al.*, (2012) conducted a meta-analysis, reviewing over 50 studies assessing victimization of children with chronic conditions, including mental health problems. Their results suggested that these children are likely to experience peer victimization. Surprisingly, their literature search revealed few studies assessing interventions to reduce bullying of children with chronic medical conditions. Increasing interactions, where abilities of children are level, between children with and without chronic illnesses was recommended as one method for improving peer acceptance of children with illnesses. Another approach was to educate peers who were developing typically about the child's condition, with the idea that improved understanding would lead to greater positive feelings toward and acceptance of the child with a medical condition. Children with mental health problems were the group least likely to experience movement toward more positive attitudes about them as a result of intervention. Sentenac *et al.*, (2012) recommended that more research with larger sample sizes and more rigorous methodological control be conducted to determine ways to improve social acceptance of children with chronic illnesses.

Sentenac *et al.*, (2011) also investigated youth reports of bullying among adolescents with disabilities and/or chronic medical conditions. Children were concerned with being bullied and younger children were more likely to report instances of bullying compared to older youth. Participants were from Ireland and

France and the authors did report that national level bully prevention efforts in France could be reducing overall rates of bullying in this country. Additionally, peer support and higher quality and more friendships were factors that could moderate the impact of and instances of bullying. As stated, the study did rely on self-report and further study assessing peers' reports of how children are treated and observational studies may yield further data to confirm study findings.

Sentenac *et al.*, (2011) and Sentenac *et al.*, (2012) took a non-categorical approach studying acceptance across a broad array of chronic conditions. On the other hand, Devine *et al.*, (2012) assessed the friendships of children with one illness, spina bifida. This chronic medical condition emerges during the first month of pregnancy when the spinal chord fails to form. A number of problems may occur, including motor paralysis, neurological difficulties, and orthopedic and urinary problems. These youth may experience social difficulties and in the study conducted by Devine *et al.*, (2012) children with spina bifida spent fewer days with friends. Conversely, they described their friendships as being close, whereas other children might not view the friendship as being very close or as close as the child with spina bifida described it to be. Children with spina bifida spent fewer days with friends and experienced lower levels of emotional support from friends. These authors recommended that interventions be conducted to improve the social skills and acceptance of children with spina bifida. Perhaps discussing the symptoms and problems associated with this chronic illness as well as teaching children who are developing typically strategies for interacting positively with children who have spina bifida would be interventions to improve their acceptance.

Although Sentenac *et al.*, (2011) and Sentenac *et al.*, (2012) used a non-categorical approach, it also is important to assess bullying, and social support, for children with different types of illnesses. Hamiwka *et al.*, (2009) studied bullying of children with epilepsy compared to their peers who were developing typically and peers with renal failure or chronic kidney disease. Their findings suggested that children with epilepsy were more likely to experience bullying compared to children who were developing typically and those with chronic kidney disease. Unexpectedly, individual or child level factors related to disease severity and social skills and depression were not related to the experience of bullying. Hence, education of peers in the classroom and in other community settings may be required and interventions to reduce bullying should target ideas for reducing bullying of children with chronic illnesses, while considering that children with some types of illness may be more likely to be bullied or "picked on" than others. Thus, mental health practitioners working in the schools should be aware that children with certain types of physical and/or cognitive limitations or children with illnesses associated with stigma may be at increased risk for peer victimization.

Emphasizing positives and strengths of the child with a chronic illness may foster his or her self-esteem and, in turn, enhance social skills and acceptance of this child. Maslow and Chung (2013) conducted a meta-analysis to review studies aimed at improving positive youth development for adolescents with a variety of chronic illnesses. The positive youth development programs stressed a positive relationship with an adult, building of leadership skills, and building positive skills for the adolescent. Many of these programs featured mentoring as a key component to improving child functioning and social skills. Helping children with chronic illnesses become aware of their own skills and assets and how to develop each of these may improve their self-esteem, which could improve their self-confidence in seeking friends. Taking a strengths-based approach to building a child's assets, including social skills, hobbies, and friendships may provide a solid social base, from which the child can confidently begin to explore his or her interests and then meet and befriend peers in his or her age range.

GRIEF REACTIONS

Children also may cope with significant grief related to their chronic illness. The course of the grief symptoms may wax and wane at different times in their development. The child may go through periods of sadness, anxiety, feelings of guilt if the child thinks his or her behavior is causing the illness, denial, and other feelings. The shifting of these feelings can be unsettling for the child and explaining the grief cycle and its stages may improve the child's understanding of what he or she is going through. The changing feelings can be described as similar to a roller coaster ride or riding one's bike down a winding hill (this can be illustrated with drawings too), so that the child can conceptualize the changing course of the grief experience. A linear model of adjustment would occur when a child moves through different stages of grief toward adjustment, without re-experiencing different stages (Worthington, 1994).

Children with chronic illness may move through more cyclical reactions to grief (Worthington, 1994), especially as they pass through different developmental stages. Consider for example, a child with facial burns. Although as a youngster the child may not feel as much sadness over the burns, when the child becomes a teenager – and enters the dating world, the facial scars may be a significant source of distress for the child. He or she may re-experience the trauma of the accident causing the burns, and feel anger associated with "missed" social opportunities if he or she is ostracized or "left out" due to stigma related to facial differences. The teenage years, thus become a developmental trigger for re-experiencing grief over a previous injury. Similar feelings may occur for other illnesses.

In other cases, "an 'event' will initiate or 'spin' the cyclical grief process." (Worthington, 1994, p. 299). Consider our previous example of the child with scars related to facial burns. If the accident occurred in fall, related to having candles burning in the home causing a fire, then fall days may remind the child of the event. The time of year in this case is a trigger. Candles may also remind the child, triggering a grief reaction. The cyclical grief pattern can also occur for other family members. Parents, for example, may re-experience their grief each year, having an "anniversary" reaction to an event related to a child's chronic medical condition. A parent may re-experience pain each year, on the eve of a child's bone marrow transplant as he or she remembers the date of the painful procedure his or her child endured. Family members who had a vision of the child leading a "normal" life, without illness or injury may be more impacted by events that could trigger the grief cycle. Worthington (1994) wrote that, "Family members who had the clearest initial vision of what the child was supposed to 'be like' may have the strongest reactions to grief-provoking events." (p. 299). Other family members, who have adjusted well to previous loss or bereavement experiences, and have a pattern of positive adjustment and moving forward after loss may, in turn, adjust relatively more easily to triggering events.

ADJUSTING TO GRIEF: WHEN COUNSELING IS ADVISABLE

Referral for therapy may be indicated if the grief reaction lasts for more than a year, without significant triggering events occurring, and if the grief reaction is intense enough to disrupt a child's or family member's ability to function in daily life activities. One technique that this author has used with children who are experiencing grief is to allow them to make a book discussing their feelings. The feelings book allows the child to review feelings in a controlled manner, as the child can, "shut the book" as needed or when he or she feels the feelings are very intense. The child has an opportunity to work through and discuss feelings and as such, has an opportunity to incorporate the illness into his or her view of the self and find meaning and new definitions for going on with life. Clark (2001) described another technique termed grief mapping, where a client would map out his or her reactions to a triggering event or condition and work through feelings to eventually arrive in a more positive place, experiencing a more positive sense of self, a new life purpose, and new meaning to life. Adjusting to grief can be a long process when a child faces a chronic illness. However, similar to Clark's (2001) notions of rebuilding life and finding purpose, a child may be reaching a more positive phase of adjustment associated with illness-related grief when he or she understands and is actively working to cope with his or her illness, finds a purpose or goals in life, and begins to build stronger social ties and a future "world" for him or herself.

ENHANCING KNOWLEDGE ABOUT CHILD THERAPY TECHNIQUES

A mental health provider interested in working with children is trained in therapeutic techniques that "work" with children. Many cognitive behavioral techniques are successful, short-term interventions for children who have chronic illnesses. A review of all possible techniques is beyond the scope of this chapter and the reader is referred to work by Kendall (2011) to begin an initial review of cognitive techniques for children. Cognitive behavioral techniques have a strong evidence base, and it is a recommended area of study, among the many areas of study, for those wishing to specialize in the treatment of children and their families. Becoming an experienced, well-versed provider is a pre-requisite for those specializing in pediatric chronic illness. Table **1** presents resources for clinicians interested in learning more about cognitive-behavioral techniques and other therapy techniques for working with children.

Table 1:   Resources for Gaining Knowledge About Cognitive-Behavioral Techniques

Book and Author(s)	Training Focus
Cognitive Therapy Techniques for Children and Adolescents: Tools for Enhancing Practice; Friedberg *et al.*	Cognitive behavioral techniques with sections that focus on "hard to reach clients".
Cognitive-Behavior Therapy for Children and Adolescents; Szigethy *et al.* (Eds.)	Cognitive and behavioral interventions with DVDs and listing of techniques in chapter appendices.
Think Good – Feel Good: A Cognitive Behavior Therapy Workbook for Children and Young People; Stellard	Worksheets based on key principles to use in therapy sessions.

Art and play therapy may be other treatment modalities for assisting a child in adjusting to grief and allowing creative outlets for emotional expression. One possible resource for clinicians is a book by Landreth *et al.,* (2005) entitled, "Play Therapy Interventions with Children's Problems: Case Studies with DSM IV-TR Diagnoses, Second Edition." Art therapy techniques that may facilitate emotional expression include "feelings masks" and paintings of "my life." A mandala of "my world" may allow the child opportunities to discuss his or her realities. These ideas are similar to some of those presented in a book entitled the, "Handbook of Art Therapy," edited by Cathy Malchiodi (2011). Medical play with toys that resemble the hospital setting may allow a child to review grief related to medical experiences in a safe and controlled setting, where he or she is in control of the hospital setting and what is happening to the characters in events that occur in this "make believe" play experience (Nabors *et al.*, 2013). Table **2** presents additional resources focusing on play therapy techniques for clinicians.

Siblings of children with chronic illnesses also may experience grief related to their brother or sister's illness. These children may require counseling to help them cope with stress related to loss of parental attention or witnessing their brother or sister cope with many painful surgeries or medical procedures. Play with medical toys may offer them opportunities to discuss their feelings if they are visiting or staying nearby and experiencing stress related to a brother or sister's hospitalization or recurrent medical procedures (Nabors *et al.*, 2013). Siblings may see the brother or sister's illness as a "family affair," such that the sibling experiences upset associated with the procedures his or her brother or sister must undergo or even sees him or herself in the sick role, so that he or she can get well or get better just like the brother or sister who actually is coping with the chronic illness. Support groups for siblings may assist them in coping with grief and trauma related to a brother or sister's illness. Similarly, brief involvement in counseling sessions, especially during times of extreme stress, such as when the child must undergo surgeries and recover from medical procedures, may assist a child in dealing with his or her feelings related to the troubles and pain his or her brother or sister is facing.

Table 2:   Resources for Play Therapy

Book and Author(s)	Training Focus
101 Favorite Play Therapy Techniques, Volume III; Kaduson & Schaefer* (Eds.)	Practical review of play therapy techniques to use during play therapy sessions.
Play Therapy: A Non-Directive Approach for Children and Adolescents: 2nd Ed.; Wilson & Ryan	Discussion of theory and review of techniques, including empathy affirmation, coping with the defiant child and use of toys.
Blending Play Therapy with Cognitive Behavioral Therapy: Evidence-based and Other Effective Treatments and Techniques; Drewes (Ed.)	Review of techniques to use with children experiencing anxiety, parent-child interaction training, and detailed protocols.

Note. *Dr. Schaefer has developed numerous books on play therapy with children.

EMOTIONAL AND BEHAVIORAL CONCERNS

Many children with chronic illnesses will function and adapt well. However, some will experience emotional and behavioral problems (Cadman *et al.*, 1987). Children experiencing problems with emotional functioning often may be experiencing symptoms of depression or anxiety at different points over the course of their illness (*e.g.*, Ramos *et al.*, 2012). Children with chronic illnesses must face the uncertainty of the waxing and waning course of their illness when illness symptoms are unpredictable, such as pain flare-ups for children with Juvenile Idiopathic Arthritis. They may feel worried about when a next episode will occur and may also feel a sense of anxiety, because they cannot control their illness.

Children with chronic pain are apt to experience feelings of stress and anxiety. Gauntlett-Gilbert *et al.*, (2013) implemented a trial of acceptance and commitment therapy with adolescents experiencing chronic pain. After participating in the treatment, adolescents reported feeling less anxious and they were more able to participate in activities. Overall, the adolescents reported that their functioning had improved as well. Participants were more accepting of their chronic illness.

Feelings of anxiety and depression can also hinder children's ability to adhere to their medical regimens. For example, Gray *et al.*, (2012) examined adolescents' perceptions of their psychological functioning and adherence. They assessed the perceptions of seventy-nine youth, between the ages of thirteen and seventeen years, who had either Crohn's Disease or Ulcerative Colitis. Participants completed measures assessing their views of their behavioral and emotional functioning and reports of barriers to adherence (such as forgetting to take medication). Ninety-six percent of the participants mentioned one or more barriers to adhering to their medical regimens. Hierarchical regression analyses were used to examine the contribution of depression and anxiety to adherence barriers. Results indicated that anxiety and depression moderated the relationship between barriers to adherence and adherence for adolescents, such that depression and anxiety had an "additive" negative impact, decreasing adherence to medical regimens. Further study, with younger children and data from parents and perhaps behavior observations will be useful in determining whether anxiety and depressive symptoms are linked in their negative impact on adherence.

One key behavioral concern for children with chronic illnesses is adhering to or following their medical regimen, although children with chronic illnesses can display a host of other types of behavioral problems. Improving their coping with their disease and its management may improve behavioral functioning and adherence to medical regimens for children with different types of illnesses (Compas *et al.*, 2012). Increasing feelings of control and efficacy for disease management may improve adherence and functioning for children and adolescents coping with illnesses. Encouraging the child to actively develop problem-solving strategies to adhere to regimens, cope with pain and disease-related problems can enhance the child's behavioral functioning as well as his or her feelings of well-being. Children and adolescents who tend to avoid coping with problems related to their illness or cope with them in an overly-emotional way, such as by feeling overwhelmed or catastrophizing and thinking of "worse" outcomes, may have more difficulty with their functioning and more emotional and behavioral problems (Compas *et al.*, 2012).

Children with chronic medical conditions are likely to experience challenges adjusting to their illness at different points in their lives. As mentioned in Chapter **1**, if the mental health provider takes a "rubber band" type of approach, and establishes an "open door" communication policy, the child and/or his or her parents can feel comfortable contacting the mental health provider when emotional and behavioral concerns arise for the child. The clinician also should be aware that he or she is treating the "whole family" and be ready to assist parents or siblings with emotional and behavioral issues. Assisting parents with coping, to be more active problem-solvers, may have positive effects on coping for the family or for the child facing and adapting to having a chronic illness (Fedele *et al.*, 2013).

Children may cope with grief reactions as they adjust to illness-related limitations, which may have different ramifications at different points in their development. For example, consider a young male with diabetes. He may not be concerned about testing his blood sugar at school, during class; however, as an adolescent he may be very concerned about testing his blood glucose level on a "date". The clinician maintains a supportive relationship so that when he or she is contacted for an "on the spot" session incidental teaching and support can occur. Moreover, teaching the child to be an active problem-solver, considering options and action steps for coping with his or her problem areas is advisable for enhancing children's coping.

EXPERIENCES WITH PEERS

Children also may feel anxious or depressed due to difficulty in their peer relationships. Children with chronic illnesses may face social isolation and ostracism or teasing and this stigma may impact emotional and behavioral functioning. They may report difficulties in peer relationships and for making friends. Some may report that they have been bullied by their peers (Van Cleave & Davis, 2006; Twyman *et al.*, 2010). These negative social experiences can have a negative impact on self-esteem and child social skills (Twyman *et al.*, 2010).

Sentenac *et al.*, (2012) assessed reports of victimization of children across several countries using a sample collected by the World Health Organization. Overall, approximately 13% of the children with chronic illnesses or disabilities in the sample mentioned they had been bullied two to three times per month. Children with disabilities were included in this sample and those with cognitive delays may have more difficulty socializing with peers and building supportive peer networks (Guralnick *et al.*, 2007). Sentenac *et al.*, (2012) found that bullying reports differed across countries. Also, results were based on self-report and thus rates of bullying could actually have been higher, especially if the children were trying to portray themselves in a positive light. Sentenac *et al.*, (2012) concluded that inclusion is a "norm" for children with chronic illnesses and that it will be important to monitor the quality of the inclusion experience and implement interventions when a child has been rejected by some peers or is having difficulty making friends.

Children with chronic illnesses may fare more positively than their peers with mental health problems and learning disabilities when it comes to experiencing ostracism. Twyman *et al.*, (2010) assessed bullying and victimization experiences for children and adolescents, aged eight to seventeen years, who were attending a routine medical visit. There were several groups: children with autism spectrum disorders, children with Attention-Deficit Hyperactivity Disorder, learning disabilities, mental health problems, and cystic fibrosis. Children with cystic fibrosis did not report significant bully-victimization experiences, whereas children with autism spectrum disorders and Attention-Deficit Hyperactivity Disorder were at increased risk for experiencing social ostracism. These researchers concluded that irrespective of type of condition, children with health care problems were at risk for experiencing ostracism. However, among the types of special health care needs, those children with cystic fibrosis appeared to face lower risks. They recommended mental health screening questions to uncover experiences of social ostracism in children with special health care needs.

Other research has indicated that some children with cancer can experience positive impacts with disease remission, such as increased feelings of self-worth and re-integration within their social networks (Wakefield *et al.*, 2010). On the other hand, they also indicated that other peers recovering from cancer still experienced negative social outcomes and negative emotional and behavioral outcomes. These children reported lower levels of well-being and feelings of self-worth as well as increased anxiety and sleeping difficulties. This seems to further support the importance of mental health screening to ensure the positive emotional, behavioral, and social functioning.

Two protective factors, which may positively impact social development, are physical skills and communication skills. Kang *et al.*, (2010) determined that youth with cerebral palsy who were better at engaging in sports and had better communication skills were more likely to be engaged in activities with peers. However, they also mentioned that changing attitudes of those in the community – to promote inclusion of children in activities – is an important intervention.[1] Assessment of protective factors – that facilitate friendships – is another area for research. Understanding child strengths related to friendships will provide information for clinicians and interventions to provide positive support to children with chronic illness.

At times, the focus of the intervention should be peers who are developing typically. Explaining the illness and positive things about the child with an illness, so that children understand and realize that they have a lot in common with the child may "open doors" to facilitate acceptance of children with chronic illnesses or disabilities. Children with chronic illnesses also interact with peers in a number of other settings, such as their neighborhoods and during after-school activities. Education of peers in these settings may improve their understanding of the child's needs so that they can include them in activities. Another idea is to assign a peer buddy to help explain the needs of and enhance the acceptance of a child with a chronic illness (Shiu, 2004).

In other instances, such as when the "target child" (the child with the chronic medical condition) is having difficulty entering play groups to interact with other children, then a possible the focus of intervention may be the child with the illness. Especially with young children, teaching group entry skills and play skills may be an intervention to improve the skills of the child so that he or she can more easily engage in interactions with peers. Alerting adults in community settings about actions and strategies to facilitate inclusion of children with chronic illnesses in social interactions and group activities is another strategy for improving chances for positive interactions for children with chronic illnesses. Furthermore, individual counseling sessions for children with chronic illnesses may be an avenue for assisting these children in developing their social skills. Adjusting activities, such as ensuring that children in wheel chairs can participate is yet another way to improve social involvement of children with chronic illnesses in activities with their peers (Shui, 2004).

In addition to considering peers as friends and supports, it remains important to "think outside the box" when considering social relationships of children with illnesses. For example, Antle *et al.*, (2009) found that children with spina bifida saw other adults as friends, such as those paid to assist them. Parents played a key role in the social worlds of many of these children. Understanding how different types of or "layers" of social support buffer children against illness-related stress as they age into young adulthood is an area for continued research. Studies of this nature will improve understanding of the nature of social support as a buffering factor throughout the early part of the lifespan.

IMPORTANCE OF PEER SUPPORT

In addition to teaching social skills to children with illnesses, the mental health professional should be prepared to educate peers about the child's condition. Education may need to occur at several system levels, including school, neighborhood, and extra-curricular activities. Children identified as bullies, who target children with medical conditions, may benefit from one-on-one counseling sessions to teach them coping skills, such as prosocial behaviors and ways to be kind to others. Other children, who are developing typically, may need to learn how to support the child with the illness, if it is a condition that may make the child more likely to be a recipient of negative peer reactions, such as epilepsy (Hamiwka *et al.*, 2009). The child with a chronic illness may feel a sense of isolation, when he or she is involved in community settings, such as school or other peer groups. This may be increased if this child has little contact with other peers who also have the same chronic illness. Assisting the child and his or her parents in finding a support group or a summer camp, where the child is able to meet peers with similar or the same medical conditions may help to reduce feelings of loneliness related to being the "only one" with a particular medical condition attending a certain school or residing in a certain neighborhood, *etc.*

Education about the child's condition is one method for improving peer support. The notion of support and acceptance of peers is critical to children's social development. Peer support is defined as, "support from a person who has experiential knowledge of a specific behavior or stressor and similar characteristics as the target population" (Hiesler, 2010, p. 124). As stated, one place where children can access this type of peer support and understanding is through attending summer camps. Woods *et al.*, (2013) evaluated outcomes for children with different types of chronic illnesses who had attended summer camp. Their findings indicated that children attending summer camps reported increased hope for accomplishing their goals and a higher quality of life. Woods *et al.*, (2013) believed that their results showed support for and were consistent with results of other studies showing that participation in summer camps increased positive social and psychological development for children with chronic illnesses.

Odar *et al.*, (2013) conducted a meta-analysis of the impact of summer camps for children with medical conditions. They reviewed 31 studies and concluded that camps had a modest positive impact on self-perceptions for some children who had chronic illnesses. Improved perceptions of the self can lead to greater self-acceptance and improved friendships (Keefe & Berndt, 1996). Thus, participation in camps, leading to improved feelings about the self can be an indirect route to increased friendships and acceptance for children with medical conditions. However, not all children attending camps experienced improved views of the self, and therefore further study of the benefits of summer camps, in terms of improved psychosocial outcomes is required.

Support groups may be another avenue for improving self-perceptions and psychosocial functioning of children with chronic illnesses. Children with illnesses, such as cancer, may benefit from peer support as well as use of technology to improve their knowledge of their disease (Zebrack & Isaacson, 2012). Facing a sense of isolation can enhance feelings of sadness for the child. Therefore, another intervention that can be effective in reducing feelings of isolation and sadness for the child is assisting the child's parents in helping the child find a support group so that he or she can connect with and reach out to peers facing similar issues. Stewart *et al.*, (2011) assessed the support needs of children with asthma and allergies and also recorded information provided by their parents. Their results demonstrated that children with asthma and allergies mentioned that they would like to meet and talk with other children with problems that were the same as or similar to their own. Their parents also saw benefit from having support from peers going through the "same thing." Kichler and her colleagues conducted psychoeducational groups for children with Type 1 Diabetes (Kichler *et al.*, 2013). These groups included education about illness and ways to improve self-management of diabetes. Groups provided children with opportunities to process key issues together, in a supportive, small group environment. Study findings did not support changes in blood glucose levels, but parents did report improved quality of life for their children. Parents also attended groups. They reported improved management of their children's diabetes. Data from studies reviewed in this paragraph represent children and adolescents in different age ranges. Research is needed to determine what specific types of supportive interventions work with youth in different age ranges. Support groups can occur at children's hospitals, online, by telephone or from joining national level organizations and attending conferences and meetings.

Online support can be beneficial for children with chronic illnesses. Nordfeldt *et al.*, (2010) assessed the impact of a portal with ideas for diabetes management and health for children with diabetes and their parents. Their evaluation results showed that participants wanted to make the portal open to others so that information about diabetes would not be a "secret." They wanted open access to information provided by health professionals and others who had diabetes. The unique support that could be obtained from peers through this internet website was thought to be valuable. Participants also reported that the information needed to be updated regularly so that it was representing cutting edge information. Making sure that information was easy to find and that the layout of the site was user-friendly was another suggestion for improving the portal. However, many of the findings in this qualitative study appeared to represent quotes from mothers using the site and more information is needed about children's views. Studies assessing child perceptions of the value of educational and supportive websites will provide knowledge to determine the value of this educational and supportive method for reaching children and providing them with access to peers facing similar situations. In a similar vein, telephone support can be another way that children with chronic illnesses could reach out to peers facing similar situations.

Heisler *et al.*, (2007) developed a model of peer support that can provide useful guidance for clinicians. They reported that peers can provide three major types of support: informational support, emotional support, and mutual reciprocity. Informational support occurs through sharing experiences with peers and learning skills, often through modeling, from peers. Emotional support is gained from being with peers who provide encouragement and help the child to feel a sense of belonging, thereby reducing feelings of isolation. Finally, mutual reciprocity occurs when children share knowledge and engage in joint problem-solving (Heisler, 2010). Peer mentoring programs, where older children, who have had the disease, advise younger children is an example of mutual reciprocity.

CASE STUDIES

Case Study 1: Boy with Apert's Syndrome

Consider the case of Zachary, a young boy with Apert's Syndrome. Children with Apert's Syndrome may have deformed or missing limbs and changes in facial features. They may also experience cognitive delays. Zachary was a preschooler having difficulty forming relationships with and interacting with peers in his classroom. He tended to interact more frequently with adults, such as teachers and student teachers. He would do "silly" things, like fall to the ground and roll to gain adult attention. These behaviors also caused his peers to avoid playing with him, both at center time in the classroom and on the playground. When adults were not with him, Zachary would often cry or sit despondently by himself in the middle of a play setting.

Interventions to improve Zachary's social interactions were threefold. First teachers and student teachers were made aware of his pattern of engaging adults in one-on-one interactions through falling on the ground. The teachers were instructed to help Zachary up and guide him to peers who were interacting. Second, Zachary was assigned a peer buddy, an older preschooler who was taught ways to play with Zachary and introduce him to play groups on the playground. Finally, Zachary received coaching in group entry skills and he learned how to ask "Can I play?" and he also learned how to join in games with mentoring from adults in the classroom. The result of this three-pronged intervention approach was increased peer interaction and reduced episodes of crying behavior. Teachers reported lower levels of depression and anxiety for Zachary.

Case Study 2: Girl with Food Allergies

Next, consider the case of Belle, an elementary school-age girl, diagnosed with allergies to mold and various trees, asthma, and Attention-Deficit Hyperactivity Disorder. She was experiencing symptoms of depression and remained isolated from peers. Her mother was concerned about her social development and emotional functioning. For Belle, interventions consisted of individual therapy to explore feelings of depression and referral for further evaluation. Belle's counselor discovered that Belle was sad because she was not able to spend time with friends outside, due to her asthma. She was also feeling depressed because she experienced peer and teacher conflict at school, as she had difficulty remaining seated, and keeping her hands to herself while waiting in line in the lunchroom.

Belle's counselor helped Belle express her feelings and discuss ideas for becoming more involved with other children. They talked about asking others how they were doing and not interrupting them, in order to begin conversations with peers. They also discussed ways to change negative thinking patterns, such as "I will never have any friends, because I can't talk to other children." Instead, Belle learned more positive self-talk, "I can ask friends about how their day is and I can talk with them." Belle responded well to identification of negative self-statements and learning and practicing positive conversation skills with peers. She also learned to more positive self-talk and to "talk-up" or talk in a positive manner about herself and her own skills. Belle noticed she was talking more with peers and they were starting to talk with her, and subsequently reported a reduction in feelings of sadness to her counselor.

Belle was referred for a medical evaluation to determine if change was needed in her medications for Attention-Deficit Hyperactivity Disorder. She had not had a medication re-evaluation in over a year. As a result of the re-evaluation, Belle's medication was slightly increased in the morning, and her ability to complete her school work improved. Belle was then able to act appropriately during class and was no longer viewed as a trouble-maker by the teacher and other students.

The counselor spent several sessions discussing involvement in extra-curricular activities that were not outside, so that Belle's allergies would not trigger the asthma episodes that interfered with her abilities to play with age peers in the neighborhood. These discussions occurred with Belle and her mother, and sometimes her father. It was decided that Belle would enroll in the "Young Scientists' Club." This was an after-school program devoted to developing children's science skills in a fun atmosphere, with peers. Science was Belle's favorite subject, so she was happy to engage in a peer group while involved in experiments in her favorite subject area. Not long after joining the group, Belle made two friends and the girls started eating lunch together and arranged "play dates" after school. As Belle's interactions with her friends increased her symptoms of depression abated. The aforementioned interventions had a positive, long-term impact on Belle's development as her symptoms of depression reduced and her functioning at school improved.

Case Study 3: Boy with Spina Bifida

Let's consider the case of Marlin, a young boy with spina bifida. His parents brought him for counseling to help him learn to cope with his chronic medical condition. Marlin's key presenting issue was, wanting to play football in the neighborhood, with older boys. Football was his favorite sport; he watched games every weekend. He wanted to be the quarterback so that he could "call the plays." Unfortunately, using a walker made it difficult for him to play on the team. Therapy offered a place for Marlin to express his feelings and problem-solve about ways to become involved on the team. Together with his therapist and parents, Marlin problem-solved and it was decided that he would meet with other boys in the neighborhood and see how he could become involved. Boys in the neighborhood were educated by Marlin's parents about the physical challenges he was facing.

The children and Marlin then met and they voted that he could be team manager and coach. He worked to arrange games and "officiate" or be a key official for the games, while at the same time acting as an advisor and helping the boys on either team develop "plays" when they had possession of the football. Marlin really enjoyed being involved in play and reported increased friendships with neighborhood boys and improved feelings of self-worth. In this manner, acceptance and support from peers was instrumental in improving Marlin's functioning in the neighborhood – a key social setting in his life. There are many other areas of a child's life where social support could be mobilized or increased. Clinicians can boost a child's resilience by developing treatment goals to improve a child's social support in key settings or contexts.

CONCLUSION

In Chapter **2**, literature related to social, emotional and behavioral problems for children and adolescents with chronic illnesses was reviewed. It was evident that children with chronic illnesses may be at risk for elevated levels of problems in the aforementioned areas. Moreover, the problems can interact, having a combined impact on child functioning. Continued training, through practica and workshop experiences, will offer clinicians alternatives for dealing with negative outcomes for youth and their families (resources in Table **1** also provide additional knowledge of therapy techniques). Alternately, children may experience grief reactions as they cope with loss related to having a chronic illness. This grief may wax and wane and be more prominent at different developmental phases. Therapeutic interventions to improve social standing and improve child self-concept may be needed at different points in the child's developmental trajectory in order to ensure acceptance and improve emotional functioning for children who have chronic illnesses. Parental involvement has the potential to improve psychosocial outcomes for children.

ACKNOWLEDGEMENTS

None declared.

CONFLICT OF INTEREST

The author confirms that this chapter contents have no conflict of interest.

REFERENCES

Antle, B. J., Montgomery, G., & Stapleford, C. (2009). The many levels of social support: Capturing the voices of young people with Spina Bifida and their parents. *Health and Social Work, 34*(2), 97-106.

Cadman, D., Boyle, M., Szatmari, P., & Offord, D. R. (1987). Chronic illness, disability, and mental and social well-being: Findings of the Ontario Child Health Study. *Pediatrics, 79*(5), 805-813.

Clark, S. (2001). Mapping grief: An active approach to grief resolution. *Death Studies, 25*, 531-548.

Compas, B. E., Jaser, S., Dunn, M. J., & Rodriguez, E. M. (2012). Coping with chronic illness in childhood and adolescence. *Annual Review of Clinical Psychology, 27*(8), 455-480.

Devine, K. A., Holmbeck, G. N., Gayes, L., & Purnell, J. Q. (2012). Friendships of children and adolescents with spina bifida: Social adjustment, social performance, and social skills. *Journal of Pediatric Psychology, 37*(2), 220-231. DOI:10.1093/jpepsy/jsr075.

Drewes, A. A. (Ed.) (2009). *Blending play therapy with cognitive behavioral therapy: Evidence-based and other effective treatments and techniques*. New York: John Wiley and Sons.

Fedele, D. A., Hullman, S. E., Chaffin, M., Kenner, C., Fisher, M. J., & Kirk, K. (2013). Impact of a parent-based intervention for mothers on adjustment in children newly diagnosed with cancer. *Journal of Pediatric Psychology, 38*(5), 531-540.

Friedberg, R. D., McClure, J. M., & Garcia, J. H. (2009). *Cognitive therapy techniques for children and adolescents: Tools for enhancing practice*. New York: Guilford Press.

Gauntlett-Gilbert, J., Connell, H., Clinch, J. & McCracken, L. M. (2013). Acceptance and values-based treatment of adolescents with chronic pain: Outcomes and their relationship to acceptance. *Journal of Pediatric Psychology, 38*(1), 72-81.

Gray, W., Denson, L. A., Baldassano, R. N., & Hommel, K. A. (2012). Treatment adherence in adolescents with inflammatory bowel disease: The collective impact of barriers to adherence and anxiety/depressive symptoms. *Journal of Pediatric Psychology, 37*(3), 282-291.

Guralnick, M. J., Neville, B., Hammond, M. A., & Connor, R. T. (2007). The friendships of young children with developmental delays: A longitudinal analysis. *Journal of Applied Developmental Psychology, 28*(1), 64-79.

Hamiwka, L. D., Yu, C. G., Haniwka, L. A., Sherman, E. M. S., Anderson, B., & Wirrell, E. (2009). Are children with epilepsy at greater risk for bullying than their peers? *Epilepsy and Behavior, 15*, 500-505.

Heisler, M. (2010). Different models to mobilize peer support to improve diabetes self-management and clinical outcomes: Evidence, logistics, evaluation consideration and needs for future research. *Family Practice, 27*, 123-132. DOI: 10.1093/fampra/cmp003.

Heisler, M., Halasyamani L, Resnicow K *et al.* (2007). ''I Am Not Alone' 'The feasibility and acceptability of Interactive Voice Response (IVR)-Facilitated Telephone Peer Support among Older Adults with Heart Failure (HF). *Congestive Heart Failure, 13*, 149–157.

Kaduson, H. G., & Schaefer, C. E. (Eds.) (2003). *101 favorite play therapy techniques: Volume III*. New York: Jason Aronson/Roman Littlefield Publishers.

Kang, L., Palisano, R., Orlin, M. N., Chiarello, L. A., King, G. A., & Polansky, M. (2010). Determinants of social participation – with friends and others who are not family members – for youths with cerebral palsy. *Physical Therapy, 90*(12), 1748-1757.

Keefe, K., & Berndt, T. J. (1996). Relations of friendship quality to self-esteem in early adolescence. *Journal of Early Adolescence, 16*, 110-129.

Kendall, P. C. (Ed.). (2011). *Child and adolescent therapy: Cognitive-behavioral procedures.* Guilford Press.

Kichler, J. C., Kaugars, A. S., Marik, P., Nabors, L., & Alemzadeh, R. (August 19, 2013, published online). Effectiveness of groups for adolescents with Type 1 Diabetes Mellitus and their parents. *Families, Systems, and Health.* No page numbers; DOI:10.1037/a0033039.

Landreth, G. L., Sweeney, D. S., Ray, D. C., Homeyer, L. E., & Glover, G. J. (2005). *Play therapy interventions with children's problems: Case studies with DSM-IV-TR Diagnoses. Second Edition.* Landham, MD: Jason Aronson and Roman and Littlefield Publishers.

Malchiodi, C. A. Edtior (2011). *Handbook of Art Therapy: Second Edition.* New York: Guilford Press.

Maslow, G. R., & Chung, R. J. (2013). Systematic review of positive youth development programs for adolescents with chronic illnesses. *Pediatrics, 131*, e1605-e1618. DOI: 10.1542/peds.2012-1615.

Nabors, L., Bartz, J., Kichler, J., Sievers, R., Elkins, R., & Pangallo, J. (2013). Play as a mechanism of working through medical trauma for children with medical illnesses and their siblings. *Issues in Comprehensive Pediatric Nursing, 36*(3), 212-224.

Nordfeldt, S., Hanberger, L., & Barterö, C. (2010). Patient and parent views on a web 2.0 diabetes portal – the management tool, generator, and the gatekeeper: Qualitative Study. *Journal of Medical Internet Research*, 12(2), e17. DOI:10.2196/jmir.1267; PMCID:PMC2956228.

Odar, C., Canter, K. S., & Roberts, M. C. (2013). Relationship between Camp Attendance and Self-Perceptions in Children with Chronic Health Conditions: A Meta-Analysis. *Journal of Pediatric Psychology*, 38(4), 398-411.

Ramos Olazagasti, M. A., Shrout, P. E., Yoshikawa, H., Bird, H. R., & Canino, G. J. (2012). The longitudinal relationship between parental reports of asthma and anxiety and depression symptoms among two groups of Peurto Rican youth. *Journal of Psychosomatic Research, 73*(4), 283-288.

Sentenac, M., Arnaud, C., Gavin, A., Molcho, M., Nic Gabhainn, S., & Godeau, E. (2012). Peer victimization among school-aged children with chronic conditions. *Epidemiological Review, 34*(1), 120-128. Doi:10.1093/epirev/mxr024.

Sentenac, M., Gavin, A., & Gabhainn, S. C. *et al.* (2012). Peer victimization and subjective health among students reporting disability or chronic illness in 11 western countries. *European Journal of Public Health, 23*(3), 421-426.

Sentenac, M., Gavin, A., Arnaud, C., Molcho, M., Godeau, E., & Gabhainn, S. N. (2011). Victims of bullying among students with a disability or chronic illness and their peers: A cross-national study between Ireland and France. *Journal of Adolescent Health, 48*, 461-466.

Shiu, S. (2004). Positive interventions for children with chronic illness: Parents' and teachers' concerns and recommendations. *Australian Journal of Education, 48*(3), 239-252.

Stellard, P. (2002). *Think good-feel good: A cognitive behavior therapy workbook for children and young people.* New York: John Wiley and Sons.

Stewart, M., Masuda, J. R., Letrouneau, N., Anderson, S., & McGhan, S. (2011). "I want to meet other kids like me": Supoort needs of children with asthma and allergies. *Issues in Comprehensive Pediatric Nursing, 34*(2), 62-78.

Szigethy, E., Weisz, J. R., & Finding, R. L. (Eds.) (2012). *Cognitive-behavior therapy for children and adolescents.* Arlington, VA: American Psychiatric Publishing.

Twyman, K. A., Saylor, C. F., Saia, D., Macias, M. M., Taylor, L. A., & Spratt, E. (2010). Bullying and ostracism experiences in children with special health care needs. *Journal of Behavioral and Developmental Pediatrics, 31*(1), 1-8.

Van Cleave, J., & Davis, M. (2006). Bullying and peer victimization among children with special health care needs. *Pediatrics, 118*(4), e1212-11219. DOI:10.1542/peds.2005-3034.

Wakefield, C. E., McLoone, J., Goodenough, B., Lenthen, K., Cairns, D. R., & Cohn, R. J. (2010). The psychosocial impact of completing childhood cancer treatment: A systematic review of the literature. *Journal of Pediatric Psychology, 35*(3), 262-274.

Wilson, K., & Ryan, V. (2005). *Play therapy: A non-directive approach for children and adolescents: Second Edition.* New York: Elsevier/Baillière Tindall.

Woods, K., Mayes, S., Bartley, E., Fedele, D., & Ryan, J. (2013). An evaluation of psychosocial outcomes for children and adolescents attending a summer camp for youth with chronic illness. *Children's Health Care, 42*(1), 85-98.

Worthington, R. C. (1994). Models of linear and cyclical grief: Different approaches to different experiences. *Clinical Pediatrics, 33*(5), 297-300.

Zebrack, B., & Isaacson, S. (2012). Psychosocial care of adolescent and young adult patients with cancer and survivors. *Journal of Clinical Oncology, 30*(11), 1221-1226.

Send Orders for Reprints to reprints@benthamscience.net

CHAPTER 3

Therapy Techniques for Assisting the Child in Coping with Mental Health Problems

Laura A. Nabors[*]

Health Education Program, School of Human Services, University of Cincinnati, 468 Dyer Hall, Mail Location 0068, Cincinnati, Ohio, OH 45221-0068, USA

Abstract: This chapter presents ideas for enhancing the emotional and behavioral functioning of children with chronic illnesses. Cognitive behavioral techniques and environmental change are reviewed as interventions commonly used in the field. Case studies, developed for use in this chapter, are used as a teaching tool, to review interventions. Three different cases are presented and these include psychotherapy or counseling for a: (1) teenager with encopresis and anxiety, (2) a boy with nut allergies, and (3) a girl with renal failure. The focus of these cases is describing interventions and the counseling process in a manner that provides ideas for various types of mental health providers working with children who have chronic illnesses.

Keywords: Anxiety, chronic illnesses, cognitive behavioral, coping orientation, depression, environmental change, therapy techniques.

INTRODUCTION

As mentioned in Chapter **2**, children with chronic illnesses are at increased risk for experiencing mental health problems. In a large-scale study, Mohler-Kuo and Day (2012) reported that about 18% of over 2,500 children in Europe who completed a screening measure had special health care needs. Of this group, over 6% required psychiatric services. Those children who were participating in mental health or psychiatric services had lower health-related quality of life and were more likely to experience behavioral problems. Children residing in low-income families with special health care needs were more likely to experience psychiatric problems. Thus, limited economic means may limit children's opportunities to

---

*Address correspondence to Laura A. Nabors:** Health Education Program, School of Human Services, University of Cincinnati, 468 Dyer Hall, Mail Location 0068, Cincinnati, Ohio, OH 45221-0068, USA; Tel: 513-556-5537; Fax: 513-556-3898; E-mail: naborsla@ucmail.uc.edu

participate in preventive mental health care or increase stress in their lives, creating increased risk for mental health problems.

Hysing *et al.*, (2009) examined the mental health of 537 children with different types of chronic illnesses. Children were placed in one of three groups for purposes of analyses: children with asthma, children with neurological disorders, and children with other types of illnesses. All three groups of children with illnesses experienced more mental health concerns than children without health care problems. Children with neurological problems had higher levels of mental health problems compared to children with asthma and children with other types of illnesses. The most common mental health problems for children with neurological concerns were difficulties with paying attention and with peer relationships.

Pinquart and Shen (2011) used a meta-analysis to examine depressive symptoms in children with different types of chronic illnesses. Over 300 studies were included in their review. Overall, they reported a higher level of depression in children experiencing illness related to healthy peers. They also found that several illness groups were at higher risk for depression. Specifically, children with cleft lip and palate, epilepsy, chronic migraine, chronic fatigue and fibromyalgia were more at risk for feeling depressed compared to children with other types of illnesses. Those in the aforementioned groups should receive monitoring and frequent evaluation of emotional functioning to rule out the experience of depressive symptoms.

ANXIETY AND DEPRESSION

Children who experience chronic illnesses or special healthcare needs often can face anxiety and as well as depression. This may be a risk for children with illnesses involving the endocrine and immune systems. Children who have chronic pain also may experience increased risk for anxiety and depression. Shelby *et al.*, (2013) studied children with chronic abdominal pain. They found that these children were at elevated risk for anxiety disorders and depression, and that this vulnerability was a long-term risk that children with chronic abdominal pain face. Others have reported that children with chronic illnesses are living longer, facing increased medical procedures and stressors related to their care, and this increase in coping with stressors may be related to increased risk for experiencing mental health problems (Halfon *et al.*, 2012). Although children with chronic illnesses face elevated risk, many children cope very well in the face of health-related stressors, chronic pain, and increased medical visits.

In a meta-analysis examining the academic, physical, and social functioning of children with chronic illnesses, Pinquart and Teubert (2012) discovered that children with chronic health concerns were more likely to face physical and social problems. Children with severe impairments also may face academic impairments, and poor functioning at school can contribute to feelings of anxiety, worry, anger, and sadness. Pinquart and Teubert (2012) mentioned that some subgroups may face elevated risk for mental health problems. Specifically, children with central nervous system limitations, such as cognitive delays, and children with more significant physical limitations related to their illnesses are at risk. Children facing cognitive and physical challenges, such as children with spina bifida and cerebral palsy, may be at increased risk for feeling isolated and experiencing academic and physical difficulties. Other chronic conditions, such as epilepsy and hearing disorders may place a child at increased risk for needing counseling related to mental health problems.

HAVING A COPING ORIENTATION

Many different therapy techniques can be successful in improving coping and involvement in daily activities for children with chronic illnesses. In broad brush strokes, it is important to outline key points for facilitating adjustment. Compas *et al.*, (2012) presented a detailed review of key factors facilitating a "coping orientation" in children with chronic illnesses. They found that active coping, involving problem-solving, environmental change, and interventions to improve child behavioral and social functioning had a positive impact on child functioning. In contrast, children focusing on negative emotions, disengaging from coping, avoiding illness-related problems, or catastrophizing (believing the worst outcomes would occur) were more likely to experience worry, sadness and emotional and behavioral problems. These problems, in turn, could be related to poor adherence to the child's medical regimen and further issues with poor health.

Interventions that facilitated a child's sense of control or an internal locus of control were likely to enhance child functioning. Disengagement or avoiding dealing with ways that illness limited life experiences and opportunities was inversely related to coping and positive functioning. Moreover, considering the child as being in a "system" of the family was important as family and parent coping had a direct impact on child coping.

Cognitive-behavioral therapy techniques – used to treat both illness-related symptoms and concomitant mental health problems can benefit children with chronic illness and co-morbid mental health problems. However, the dual benefit of treating illness symptoms and mental health problems is not always realized. For example, Palermo *et al.*, (2010) conducted a meta-analysis and reported that cognitive-behavioral treatments, such as relaxation and exposure therapies were effective in the treatment chronic pain in children, but did not necessarily always result in improvements in mental health symptoms.

However, in general many clinicians utilize cognitive-behavioral therapies and other modes of psychotherapy to successfully work with children with chronic illnesses and co-occurring mental health problems. There are several good resources for cognitive-behavioral therapy treatment of children with mental health concerns. Resources for treatment can be found in several textbooks including one edited by Kendall (2011) and another edited by Graham and Reynolds (2013). Many different resources exist for practitioners and thus the goal of this chapter is to educate about treatment using case examples to directly illustrate some ideas for treatment of children with co-morbid chronic illness and mental health issues.

RECOMMENDED JOURNALS

Several journals provide a compilation of treatment techniques that improve disease-related problems, such as pain and psychological problems in children and adolescent with chronic illnesses. One journal of interest is the *Journal of Pediatric Psychology*. Others include: *Child: Health, Care, and Development*, the *Journal of Developmental and Behavioral Pediatrics*, *Pediatrics*, and *Clinical Practice in Pediatric Psychology*. There are many other outlets for learning of therapy that is effective in assisting children with chronic illnesses. A hallmark educational text, which was mentioned earlier is, the *Handbook of Pediatric Psychology* (Roberts & Steele, 2009). Specialized training, in hospitals and with experts who have worked with children with health problems is recommended, in addition to extensive education in the field, to assist those who wish to specialize in mental health treatment for children with chronic health problems.

With the aforementioned factors in mind, one has a general picture of factors the either facilitate or detract from child coping. Positively changing the child's environment, providing a supportive therapy environment for the child to release feelings and brain-storm or problem- solve, as well as encouraging the child to increase feelings of personal control over disease management can improve child functioning. In general, facilitating positive, action-oriented strategies are of benefit to improving child feelings of personal control and commitment to managing disease. Providing positive statements and praise to improve the child's feelings about him- or herself can lead to improved feelings of self-worth and personal efficacy for illness management. The following cases present ideas of therapy techniques that enhanced coping. Table **1** presents a review of techniques that this author has found helpful in working with children with chronic illness and their families, when consulting in hospital and private practice settings.

Table 1:   **Therapy Techniques for Children with Medical Conditions for Three Case Studies**

Case	Techniques Reviewed	References
Girl with retentive encopresis and trichotillomania	Importance of positive self-regard and positive self-statements; contracts to improve adherence to regimen and honest reporting of medical problems; increasing parent-child communication; psycho-education regarding medical condition and importance of high fiber diet; preventing negative behaviors (hair-pulling) and substitution of positive behaviors.	McGrath *et al.*, (2000); Nabors and Morgan (1995); Tomkins (2014); Vitulano *et al.*, (1992)
Boy with medical fears related to nut allergies	Empathic listening with acceptance of the child through play, desensitization procedures, anxiety management strategies, modeling for parent.	Axline (1969); Beidel and Alfano (2013); Crenshaw and Kenney-Noziska (2013); Flatt and King (2010); Uman *et al.*, (2013)
Girl with renal failure	Play therapy with unconditional positive regard for the child; networking and education with mother and medical team; psycho-education about dietary needs for children with renal disease.	Axline (1969); Drotar (2013); Keller and Sarvet (2013); Swallow *et al.*, (2013)

Three case studies, with review of interventions mentioned in Table **1**, are presented to illustrate the intervention with children who have chronic illnesses. The three cases focus on a teenage girl with retentive encopresis and trichotillomania, a boy with medical fears and nut allergies, and a girl experiencing renal failure. Extensive information is presented in case studies to provide the reader with a depth view of interventions and treatment.

CASE STUDIES

Case Study 1: Girl with Retentive Encopresis and Trichotillomania

Rayma was a teenager with recurrent anxiety and depression related to chronic constipation, and subsequent retentive encopresis. Rayma had been coping with encopresis since early elementary school. She had undergone multiple medical procedures to "clean out" her system. She struggled with aganglionic megacolon, as chronic constipation had stretched her colon, such that was difficult for her to feel the urge to go to the bathroom. Rayma was referred to counseling by her mother and pediatrician during her 8th grade school year. Her mother and pediatrician noted increasing problems with academic performance and socialization. Rayma was staying home more often, began pulling out her hair, and was avoiding interactions with family and peers. Her grades had fallen as well.

After a detailed interview with Rayma and her mother, she was diagnosed with trichotillomania and the specialist she had seen at a nearby pediatric hospital had previously diagnosed her with encopresis. Rayma was sad and cried when discussing her gastrointestinal problems which she believed, "I will never be rid of." She perceived herself in a negative fashion due to her encopresis and frequent accidents that she was continually trying to hide. She did not have a sense that her condition would improve and she worried the "worst" would happen-- that she would have a hospital stay and procedures related to her encopresis. When she began pondering these negative outcomes and thinking about problems with relating to peers during the school day, she would pull her hair out. This typically occurred before she fell asleep each night.

Rayma had a tendency to "catastrophize" or expect the worst possible outcomes related to health issues. She felt little control over her current health problems and felt that they happened "to" her and she had no control in working to improve her physical symptoms. Several sessions were needed to build rapport and the mental health professional focused on "listening" to Rayma. As Rayma told stories about home, she seemed to indicate that she needed more attention from her mother and that she was suffering from negative comments made by her younger brother about her "bathroom problems." She also felt distanced from her father, who often avoided her because he felt guilty because Rayma had "inherited" his medical problems. Her father would not attend counseling sessions, because he did not believe in therapy. Counseling thus focused on working with Rayma and her mother.

Several interventions were implemented to help Rayma increase her knowledge about and coping with her encopresis. Rayma learned, through psychoeducational sessions, about the importance of drinking water and other liquids, and consuming foods that were higher in fiber. She learned she liked wheat bread and fiber bars, which helped her condition. She developed behavioral contracts with the therapist to take her mineral oil, prescribed by her doctor, every other day. She was supposed to consume mineral oil each day, but would not agree to this. But, with contracting and a reward system, the prize was going out to eat with her mother, Rayma was able to begin to take her medicine every other day.

Rayma also charted her most likely time to have accidents, which was in the afternoon. This lead to home and school-based environmental interventions so that Rayma could use the bathroom at the time during which accidents were likely to occur. After identifying higher fiber foods she liked to eat with her therapist, Rayma also was able to begin to monitor and chart her food consumption and she found that drinking more water and eating higher fiber foods was improving her ability to use the bathroom to relieve constipation.

Rayma had found her condition overwhelming and was avoiding telling her mother and others about her accidents by hiding her panties in a bag under her bed. Her parents had found her bag and this lead to conflict between her and them, as Rayma's parents felt she was not being honest with them. Rayma learned, through role play and practice in therapy sessions, to communicate with her mother about her accidents. Then, in the supportive environment, she requested sessions with her mother to talk about being able to spend time with her mother discussing planning regarding diet and ways to deal with her condition. She ended up mentioning that her brother was teasing her about her accidents and she became very tearful when discussing his behavior. She and her mother worked out a secret signal (thumbs up sign) to indicate that she might need to discuss her encopresis management with her mother, without her brother being present. Her mother also had several "talks" with her brother to explain the impact of his teasing and help him learn not to tease his sister about her encopresis. Both of the aforementioned interventions resulted in improved feelings of being able to control her illness or exert an impact on illness management and feelings of anxiety and depression reduced.

Rayma's teacher was informed about her "afternoon" accidents. She was understanding and agreed to provide Rayma with a pass to the restroom during the afternoon. The school nurse also became involved and kept extra panties in her office for Rayma to use if an accident occurred. Rayma became less anxious about going to school and after time was observed to socialize more with peers.

Rayma showed improved adherence to drinking more liquids and eating more high fiber foods. Her constipation decreased and she had long periods of time when she did not experience leakage or accidents related to her encopresis. She had several positive interactions with her GI doctor, which improved their relationship and further elevated her confidence for adhering to medical instructions and being able to play a key role in working through problems related to her illness.

Behavioral interventions, involving response prevention, were used to tackle hair pulling. Also, environmental changes, such as removing her bunk bed and getting her a larger, queen-sized bed that stayed on the ground reduced feelings of nervousness related to sleeping "too high up" from the ground. Rayma also wore gloves to bed -- thick work gloves -- and she did not pull her hair when wearing the gloves. At first she resisted wearing the gloves, because they felt "different and strange." Her mother agreed to monitor her putting on gloves at bedtime.

Also, in joint therapy sessions, Rayma, her mother and the therapist worked to develop a reward chart so that Rayma could receive reinforcement for wearing gloves all night long.

About 2 weeks after wearing gloves, and changing her bed to one on the floor, Rayma and her mother reported she was only hair pulling when she did not wear her gloves to bed. Some hair had started to grow in, which was very exciting for both women, as school was going to start, and Rayma was embarrassed about having thinning hair at various places on her head. She and her mother purchased hair bands and pony tail holders to pull her hair over thinning spots. Her father, who was discussing keeping her home from school if she continued to pull out her hair, agreed to a telephone session with the therapist.

During this session they discussed his concerns and wanting to protect his daughter by keeping her home if she looked different due to her hair pulling. After he had expressed feelings, the therapist talked to him about how much his daughter wanted to go to school and be with her peers. She also shared that his daughter had reported that her father's continued upset feelings related to her hair pulling were making her feel very anxious and putting her at risk for pulling her hair because she was anxious when she went to bed. Her father agreed to stop talking about staying home from school and to engage in positive conversations with his daughter -- that involved positive things she was accomplishing rather than focusing on her problems. This lead to an improvement in their relationship. Rayma stopped pulling her hair and the behavior chart and eventually the gloves were no longer needed.

Simultaneously, Rayma became more involved in school activities, joining the young writers' club and the mad scientists' club. She made two new friends through these activities, which further improved feelings of self-worth and anxiety and sadness reduced. Moreover, lying about accidents had stopped and Rayma was willing to practice going to the bathroom on the toilet when she came home from school. Thus, several interventions including education, support, response prevention, environmental change, behavioral contracting, reinforcement, and family therapy sessions were supports to improving child functioning.

Case 2: Boy with Medical Fears Related to Severe Nut Allergies

Douglass was a 5-year-old boy with severe nut allergies. He was allergic to all kinds of nuts, especially pine nuts. This was discovered when he was in preschool and had a peanut butter cracker at daycare. His tongue and throat swelled. He had difficulty breathing after taking a few bites of the peanut butter cracker. His teacher called his mother, who luckily was home, and his mother rushed Douglass to the local children's hospital emergency room.

Upon entering the emergency room, staff was immediately in attendance and reported he needed emergency treatment. He was rushed to a room where an epi-pen was produced and he was given a shot. He was afraid of the needle and moved and consequently the first shot did not work. Unfortunately, he had to have a second one. At this point, Douglass was very scared and members of the medical team had to hold him down to administer the epi-pen. This shot did work, but Douglass was left traumatized from his first emergency room experience.

After this, Douglass became fearful of any type of nut, even if it was a child eating a nut or peanut butter sandwich several tables away from him at school (he ate at the nut free table) or if he saw a picture or pictures of various types of nuts. Douglass would not attend events at friends' homes and he would not go on "play dates" away from home due to fears that he might come in contact with peanuts. His fears were limiting his social life and limiting the family's engagement as a group, as there were events they could not attend because Douglass would become upset for fear of coming into contact with a peanut. Douglass had developed a phobia related to his medical condition.

Counseling involved a process of desensitization as well as education to teach Douglass anxiety management skills. Therapeutic rapport was established in preliminary sessions. Then, Douglass began learning strategies to manage worry, including muscle relaxation, imagining positive events (like his birthday party or going on vacation), distraction (doing something fun when feeling nervous), and using logic by "talking back to worries" by telling them that they were not likely to happen and were taking away from his "fun" time. Douglass's favorite strategy was muscle relaxation -- the rock sponge activity. During this exercise he clenched and unclenched his fists and feet to release worries (*i.e.*, body tension) related to nut fears. He also learned to combine muscle relaxing with talking back to his worries to tell them that they were "overdoing it" and needed to "shrink down and away."

After Douglass had good skills using his worry strategies and was having reduced worry about eating lunch at school, the therapist and his mother conversed about using reward charts at home for times when he was able to look at a book with nuts in it. The reward Douglass selected was to play games with his mother or father each time he could look at a picture in the book without crying.

After 2 weeks, Douglass had earned lots of "game time" with his parents and he was able to look at 4 pages of the book with pictures of how to cook with nuts without crying and becoming upset. He had found that a challenge strategy, where he said, "Worries you are silly," was helping him to defeat negative and anxiety provoking thoughts about having a reaction to seeing a picture of a nut. His biggest fear was having a reaction and going to the hospital. Therapy sessions focused on allowing him to process this fear and educating him about how the epi-pen would always protect him. Positive self-talk and talking about steps for staying safe seemed to have a calming effect for Douglass. He learned to discuss his fear and realize that the possibility of having a severe allergic reaction was greatly reduced with the medical plans and solutions that were in place.

Douglass benefitted greatly from talking about worries and learning strategies. The therapist, in consultation with his mother, decided to attempt a systematic desensitization procedure, in order to further reduce nut-related anxiety (Rimm & Masters, 1979). Systematic desensitization was developed by Joseph Wolpe to reduce phobic reactions. Douglass began the desensitization process by developing an anxiety hierarchy with the therapist. He discussed all the situations that made him nervous. Douglass and his therapist drew pictures of each situation on note cards. Then, over two sessions, they worked to arrange the pictures from lowest to highest, in terms of their anxiety-provoking potential. Douglass worked through his hierarchy slowly taking "play breaks" whenever he needed them or became nervous about making pictures of things that worried or scared him about his nut allergy. During these same sessions, Douglass and his therapist decided upon relaxation strategies that would be the "best" ones to calm him if Douglass viewed one of the pictures in his hierarchy. Douglass decided that muscle relaxation, in combination with telling his worries to, "Go down, because it will be OK." was a favorite strategy.

At a third session, the therapist explained to Douglass that they would discuss the anxiety cards and that he would relax his way through his feelings so that he no longer felt nervous, worried or scared about the card. They talked about using his strategies to calm down and to signal the therapist with a "thumbs up" sign when he was no longer scared about the situation in the card. After this, he would play games and with toys for a bit. Then, they would review another card in his anxiety hierarchy. To construct the anxiety hierarchy cards were ordered from the one that produced the lowest level of upset and anxious feelings to the one that produced the highest level of upset and anxious feelings.

Over a series of three more sessions, Douglass and his therapist reviewed all the cards and he "relaxed his way" through feelings of worry related to each situation depicted in a card. Douglass also used a stop signal -- putting up is hand in a "stop" gesture, to stop the desensitization procedure if a card was making him nervous. He and the therapist made sure he was relaxed when going through each level of the hierarchy and he always ended his sessions on a positive experience working through a card in his hierarchy. At the end of the third session he had worked through the cards. Douglass was very excited with his success in moving through his anxiety hierarchy. His mother reported that Douglass was talking less about his nut allergies at home and had agreed to go on a play date at a friend's home. The play session went very well and after another few weeks, he was invited to and attended a birthday party at a friend's house. As successes continued to build, Douglass talked less about his fears, expressed lower levels of fear, and was able to re-engage in typical activities for a child his age.

Douglass was able to successfully review his fear hierarchy two more times in counseling sessions and then he was able to go through his hierarchy, relaxing when needed, with his mother at home. His worries decreased and he was able to stay at his lunch table when another child in the room ate a peanut butter sandwich at the table next to him. Douglass's mother was pleased with his progress. She believed he would be calm and able to assist, and not become upset and combative, should he need to use the epi-pen if he ingested or came into contact with nuts. Consequently, a variety of supportive, educational, and cognitive-behavioral interventions were utilized to improve coping and increase social involvement and sense of personal control for this young child with fears related to his nut allergies.

There are times when psychotherapy for mental health problems is rejected by children with chronic illnesses, because they attribute their feelings of sadness solely to disease processes. For instance, this author has worked with several adolescents with recurrent bowel pain who attributed symptoms of depression to the waxing and waning course of their illness. Because of involvement in many medical visits to treat gastrointestinal problems and because they believed the feelings of depression would pass when their disease resolved, these adolescents declined to participate in counseling. This occurred despite urging by their parents and doctors or medical care team. Therapists and counselors should strive to build rapport and offer to be available when needed in order to try to engage these reluctant clients in counseling. It may be the case that the child is in denial of mental health problems and having an "open door" policy and working to establish a helping relationship can facilitate conditions whereby the youth will seek treatment for symptoms of depression or other mental health concerns. Moreover, the medical care team may refer these youth to support groups with peers with similar chronic illnesses, in the hopes that counselors leading these groups can form therapeutic relationships so that the youth may become comfortable addressing emotional problems.

Case 3: Girl Experiencing Renal Failure

Renee was a seven-year-old girl experiencing renal failure and waiting for a kidney transplant. She received dialysis three days per week. Her adherence to her medical regimen, in terms of reducing intake of liquids, especially on weekends where there was an extra day between dialysis treatments, was very poor. She would often sneak food, especially Watermelon and fruit juices, which were her favorite snacks. This made her retain water and she was bloated and uncomfortable when coming for dialysis treatment on Mondays. Renee had become depressed while waiting for her kidney transplant. She was often uncommunicative while receiving dialysis treatments. Her mother, a single parent with two jobs, did not have "leave" time to take Renee to counseling sessions. Moreover, her mother had very poor abilities to monitor food intake of the children at home, so it was often the case that Renee was eating foods that were high in salt content and having too much fluid.

The team at the dialysis center had become so concerned about Renee's adherence to diet and liquid intake that the nurses had contacted social services reporting "neglect" of medical care was occurring in the home. A social services worker had investigated the conditions at home, issued a warning to Renee's mother to be more vigilant, and then the case was dropped. The mother was not cited nor were there any follow-up visits to monitor dietary adherence in the home. The mother was significantly angered by the report and believed that the nurses in the dialysis unit had made a call to report her, although no one in the unit had ever admitted to this and the report was confidential in nature. Hence, relations between the mother and the medical team were strained, such that any recommendations about Renee's welfare by the medical team, including discussion of her being sad and depressed, were ignored by Renee's mother or dismissed as "unfounded."

The nurses and attending physician made a referral to the pediatric psychologist. The mother met with the pediatric psychologist at the urging of the medical team and reluctantly agreed to counseling – but only during the time that Renee was receiving dialysis and "had nothing else to do." The therapist began visiting Renee when she was receiving dialysis. At first, Renee was uncommunicative, and she pretended that the therapist was "not there." She looked at others, but would not make eye contact with or talk with the therapist. After two visits, the therapist began bringing books and toys and played "alongside" Renee as she received her dialysis treatments. At the third visit, Renee reached for the toys. During this visit and the next, she played with the toys alone, and avoided contact with the therapist. By the fifth visit, Renee made eye contact and asked for toys to play with. The toys were medical toys – hospital beds and small figures representing patients and doctors. She also asked for other toys the therapist had brought, including paper dolls and clothes as well as a Cush ball and crayons and paper. She played with all the toys and mumbled thanks as the therapist left. The therapist introduced herself and said she had enjoyed watching Renee play.

During session six, the therapist introduced herself as she handed Renee the toys and asked Renee how she was doing. Renee replied, "O.K." They played side-by-side at the beginning of the session and by the end of the session were engaging in interactive play where they conversed about play scenarios. They discussed a medical situation with the small figures and the medical toys where a child would receive surgery and then "get well." Then, the child would be able to be with her family "all the time." After more play sessions, Renee was able to talk with the therapist without the dolls and talk about her sadness related to her dialysis and her kidney failure. She did not like the diet, and especially did not care for fluid restrictions as she loved soda. Over time, Renee was able to discuss her sad feelings and her feelings of helplessness as she waited to receive a kidney. She also talked about feeling sad because her mother was not home very much, because she had to work two jobs to support their small family. After several sessions, it was noted that Renee was restricting her fluid access and that her health had improved. Renee seemed to benefit from expressing her feelings about missing her mother and worrying about her mother. After talking about her feelings she appeared relieved. The supportive nature of play therapy thus can be another avenue for helping children cope with illness. One journal that may be of value to practitioners is the *International Journal of Play Therapy* and learning about play therapy through supervision and education is another avenue for learning therapy techniques that can be useful for children. Clark (1998, 2003) has written about the healing nature of play as an avenue for enhancing coping and adjustment of children with chronic illnesses. She has assessed children's use of play to express emotional concerns as well as promote their healing and expression of hopes for the future.

CONCLUSION

As discussed at the beginning of this chapter, children with chronic health conditions or chronic illnesses can face behavioral and emotional problems related to their health concerns. Referral for counseling to help them learn strategies for overcoming worries and strategies to improve skills in disease management can be an important ancillary service for improving child coping with illness as well as child psychosocial functioning. Interventions to improve social involvement, change environmental barriers, gain support from family members, and improve child feelings of efficacy for disease management are tools of the trade for assisting children in coping with illness-related stress, anxiety, depression or behavioral concerns.

ACKNOWLEDGEMENTS

None declared.

CONFLICT OF INTEREST

The author confirms that this chapter contents have no conflict of interest.

REFERENCES

Axline, V. M. (1969). *Play therapy*. New York: Ballantine Books.

Beidel, D. C., & Alfano, C. A. (2013). *Child anxiety disorders: A guide to research and treatment: Second Edition*. New York: Taylor & Francis.

Clark, C. D. (1998). Childhood imagination in the face of chronic illness. In J. de Rivera & T. R. Sarbin (Eds). *Believed-in imaginings: The narrative construction of reality: Memory, trauma, dissociation, and hypnosis series* (pp. 87-100). Washington, D. C.: American Psychological Association.

Clark, C. D. (2003). *In sickness and in play: Children coping with chronic illness*. Brunswick, N.J.: Rutgers University Press.

Compas, B. E., Jaser, S., Dunn, M. J., & Rodriguez, E. M. (2012). Coping with chronic illness in childhood and adolescence. *Annual Review of Clinical Psychology, 27*(8), 455-480.

Crenshaw, D. A., & Kenney-Noziska, S. (2014). Therapeutic presence in play therapy. *International Journal of Play Therapy*, *23*(1), 31-43.

Drotar, D. (2013). Reflections on clinical practice in pediatric psychology and implications for the field. *Clinical Practice in Pediatric Psychology*, *1*(2), 95-105.

Flatt, N., & King, N. (2010). Brief psycho-social interventions in the treatment of specific childhood phobias: a controlled trial and a 1-year follow-up. *Behaviour Change, 27*(3), 130-153.

Graham, P., & Reynolds, S. Eds. (2013). *Cognitive behavioral therapy for children and families. Third Edition*. New York: Cambridge University Press.

Halfon, N., Houtrow, A., Larson, K. & Newacheck, D. W. (2012). The changing landscape of disability in childhood. *The Future of Children, 22*(1), 13-42.

Hysing, M., Elgen, I., Gillberg, C., & Lundervold, A. J. (2009). Emotional and behavioral problems in subgroups of children with chronic illness: Results from a large-scale population study. *Child: Care, Health and Development, 35*(4), 527-533.

Keller, D., & Sarvet, B. (2013). Is there a psychiatrist in the house? Integrating child psychiatry into the pediatric medical home. *Journal of the American Academy of Child and Adolescent Psychiatry, 52*(1), 3-5.

Kendall, P. C., Ed. (2011). *Child and adolescent therapy: Cognitive Behavioral Procedures. Fourth Edition.* New York: Guilford Press.

McGrath, M. L., Mellon, M. W., & Murphy, L. (2000). Empirically supported treatments in pediatric psychology: Constipation and encopresis. *Journal of Pediatric Psychology, 25*(4), 225-254.

Mohler-Kuo, M., & Day, M. (2012). A comparison of health-related quality of life between children with *versus* without special health care needs, and children requiring *versus* not requiring psychiatric services. *Quality of Life Research, 21*(9), 1577-1586.

Nabors, L., & Morgan, S. B. (1995). Treating retentive encopresis: Dietary modification and behavioral techniques. *Child and Family Behavior Therapy, 17*(1), 47-58.

Palermo, T. M., Eccleston, C., Lewandowski, A. S., Williams, A. C., & Morley, S. (2010). Randomized controlled trials of psychological therapies for management of chronic pain in children and adolescents: An updated meta-analytic review. *Pain, 148*(3), 387-397.

Pinquart, M., & Teubert, D. (2012). Academic, physical, and social functioning of children and adolescents with chronic physical illness: A meta-analysis. *Journal of Pediatric Psychology, 37*(4), 376-389.

Pinquart, M., & Shen, Y. (2011). Depressive symptoms in children and adolescents with chronic physical illness: An updated meta-analysis. *Journal of Pediatric Psychology, 36*(4), 375-384.

Rimm, D. C., & Masters, J. C. (1979). *Behavior therapy: Techniques and empirical findings. Second Edition.* New York: Academic Press.

Roberts, M. C., & Steele, R. G. Eds. (2009). *Handbook of pediatric psychology: Fourth edition.* New York: Guilford Press.

Shelby, G. D., Shirkey, K. C., Sherman, A. L., Beck, J. E., Haman, K., Shears, A. R., *et al.* (2013). Functional abdominal pain in childhood and long-term vulnerability to anxiety disorders. *Pediatrics, 132*(3), 475-482. DOI:10.1542/peds 2012-2191.

Swallow, V. M., Nightingale, R., Williams, J., Lambert, H., Webb, N. J., Smith, T., ... & Allen, D. (2013). Multidisciplinary teams, and parents, negotiating common ground in shared-care of children with long-term conditions: A mixed methods study. *British Medical Care: Health Services Research, 13*(1), 1-17.

Tompkins, M. A. (2014). Cognitive–behavior therapy for pediatric trichotillomania. *Journal of Rational-Emotive & Cognitive-Behavior Therapy, 32*, 98-109.

Uman, L. S., Birnie, K. A., Noel, M., Parker, J. A., Chambers, C. T., McGrath, P. J., & Kisely, S. R. (2013). Psychological interventions for needle-related procedural pain and distress in children and adolescents. *Cochrane Database Systematic Review, 10*. John Wiley and Sons.

Vitulano, L. A., King, R. A., Scahill, L., & Cohen, D. J. (1992). Behavioral treatment of children and adolescents with trichotillomania. *Journal of the American Academy of Child and Adolescent Psychiatry, 31*(1), 139-146.

CHAPTER 4

Care Plans in the School Setting

Laura A. Nabors[*]

Health Education Program, School of Human Services, University of Cincinnati, 468 Dyer Hall, Mail Location 0068, Cincinnati, Ohio, OH 45221-0068, USA

Abstract: This chapter introduces the idea of developing written care plans to assist school personnel in learning about how to intervene and handle child chronic illnesses in the school setting. Critical components of care plans, including ideas for emergency planning, are reviewed. In addition, resources for teachers, ideas for improving collaboration and communication with teachers, and ideas for working with schools are presented. School reintegration after an extended hospital stay can be challenging and research highlighting ways to make school re-entry successful are delineated. Case studies, with outlines of school care plans and interventions, are presented at the end of the chapter.

Keywords: Care plans, educational planning, emergency planning, school functioning, school reintegration, teacher training.

INTRODUCTION

Children with chronic illnesses often benefit from planning to assist them in managing their illness at school. This setting is an important social setting for children and adolescents, and thus keeping in mind that they are observed by their peers is an important part of school-based care planning. Some children may require Individual Education Plans, whereas others may require only emergency care planning. Children with chronic illnesses can benefit from Section 504 plans to help assist them in meeting their health care needs in the school setting. Children with Section 504 plans are considered "other health impaired." This type of special education designation can provide a mechanism for documenting the child's health problems and planning for assisting the child during the school day

---

*Address correspondence to Laura A. Nabors:** Health Education Program, School of Human Services, University of Cincinnati, 468 Dyer Hall, Mail Location 0068, Cincinnati, Ohio, OH 45221-0068, USA; Tel: 513-556-5537; Fax: 513-556-3898; E-mail: naborsla@ucmail.uc.edu

and during after-school activities. These plans can be broad ranging – from ensuring that young children with arthritis receive an extra set of books and a pass to use the school elevator when they are experiencing an arthritis flare-up to allowing children with diabetes an option to test their blood sugar whenever necessary and to keep snacks with them in the classroom. Section 504 plans and other types of special education planning can be very helpful to children with special health care needs and at the same time can educate school staff about the child's concerns, needs, and medical regimen.

The mental health provider can serve as a liaison for the child when developing special health care plans for the school setting. In this role, one task is to open lines of communication between the health care team and school staff, so that they can communicate about the child's health and progress. In a "connecting" type of role, the mental health provider can also transmit information from the child's medical team to the child's teacher and school nurse. Many schools do not have full-time nursing care. This may be something that the mental health provider needs to advocate for. Ensuring that others are trained in health care provision, such as the use of inhalers for children with asthma, if a nurse is not present during the school day is another important goal. It is advisable to have daily care plans and emergency plans in writing. Teachers should also be aware of the child's emergency medical contacts and any instructions for contacting the child's medical team or parents in an emergency situation.

DEVELOPING CARE PLANS

There are many important areas to include in a child's care plan. Some ideas to consider are: (1) emergency preparedness training; (2) steps for coping in any type of medically-related emergency care situation; (3) ideas and "steps" for helping the child engage in interactions during recess, lunch, and during class time; (4) steps for assisting the child in participating in recreational and extra-curricular activities; (5) nutritional planning; (6) ideas for improving social involvement; and (7) ideas for assistance the child needs in completing class work (Nabors *et al.*, 2012). The aforementioned list is a starting point for working in schools and is by no means an exhaustive list. Care plans also should have a section ensuring that the school is aware of the need to help the child "make up" or complete any missed assignments due to doctor's visits or hospitalizations. When children face longer hospital stays, plans for tutoring and delivery of assignments are necessary components of care planning. When some children return from a hospital stay, special planning for their reintegration into the classroom and involvement in the daily school routine may be needed.

Table **1** presents a list of key areas to include in care plans for children with special needs.

Table 1:   Ideas for Health Care Plans

Specifics about the medical condition
Ideas for care of the condition in the classroom (routine care and special issues)
What to do on field trips
Ideas for meeting the child's needs during special classes, such as music, art, physical education
Plans for extra-curricular activities
What to do if the nurse is absent
Instructions for working with the school nurse
Parent contacts
Specific needs: (1) nutrition, (2) physical activity, (3) peers, and (4) behavior management
Educational planning
Emergency contacts
Emergency situation description and instructions for care
Plans for school absences
Reintegration planning

It is noteworthy that the emergency care plan is subsumed in the school care plan. However, this is such an important issue that the emergency care plan may be a separate document that is carefully reviewed with teachers and the school nurse as well as other relevant school professionals (see Table **1**).

Communication between the medical team and school may be a challenge (Nolan *et al.*, 2007). Including a representative from the child's medical team in meetings can ensure that their input drives school planning. A thorough assessment of child's cognitive, social, behavioral, and emotional functioning is recommended and the mental health provider can play a key role in conducting these assessments. The school nurse or school district's nurse is another key player to include in the development and implementation of care plans. The school nurse can serve as a "point person" in developing care plans in consultation with members of the medical team. In addition, it may be useful to identify a case manager from among school staff to manage and update the child's care plan. The interval for updating the plan should be established when the plan is created.

Developing a system of medication administration for children can ease stress related to taking medications, which can be difficult to administer in the school setting (Smith *et al.*, 2008). The American Academy of Pediatrics, Council on School Health (2009), has developed guidelines for administration of medications in schools. The case manager for the child's care plan can periodically check and ensure that medication administration is running smoothly. Establishing a connection with the medical team can also provide a conduit for learning about changes in medication management.

Children with chronic medical conditions may miss opportunities to be involved in extracurricular activities, such as sports and band (Nabors *et al.*, 2012). The mental health provider is in an optimal position to work with parents and the medical team to develop plans to maximize child participation in extracurricular activities – written plans for child involvement in after-school activities, tutoring for group leaders and coaches is recommended. Furthermore, writing down the plan and submitting a copy, with emergency contacts, to leaders of after-school programs can reduce their feelings of concern and doubt over best practices in caring for the child. The coach or leader can write down emergency contacts and planning information on a note card to keep available during off-campus extracurricular activities. An emergency card may also be beneficial for teachers to carry when on field trips.

MODEL FOR SCHOOL PLANNING

The "4D" model is a method for guiding planning and continuous evaluation of the child's care plan (Forrest *et al.,* 1997). A primary consideration is continuous monitoring of the child's cognitive, emotional, and physical development. As the child develops changes in cognitive abilities may occur, especially if the child is receiving treatments that may impact cognitive functioning, such as chemotherapy, or have a disease that can be related to cognitive change, such as HIV. The mental health provider can help the school team by understanding the parent-child relationship, particularly in regard to its impact on the child's abilities for self-management of his or her medical condition (DeWalt & Hink, 2009). The mental health provider also should be knowledgeable about the differential courses of illness in children compared to adults. This includes recognition of how the timing of a chronic illness may affect the cognitive development and the psychosocial correlates of the disease. Mental health providers and the school team need to consider "culture," and they need to develop culturally and linguistically sensitive approaches to enhancing the health literacy of the child and family (DeWalt & Hink, 2009).

EDUCATIONAL PLANNING

Developing a plan using the Section 504 label of "other health impaired" can be beneficial. Detailed information about 504 plans is also presented in Chapter **5**. The American Diabetes Association (2004) developed a good example of a school plan that highlights ideas about childhood diabetes, but it can be modified and serves as a template for a section 504 plan for other types of childhood chronic illnesses. If parents or professionals need further information about the basic rights of persons with chronic medical conditions I recommend a book by Jaff (2010) entitled, "Know Your Rights: A Handbook for Patients with a Chronic Illness." The ideas addressed in the school plan should be similar to those outlined in Table **1**. The mental health provider can assist in the development of a written plan and can provide support for the child by (1) identifying barriers to forming positive relationships with peers (Vance & Eiser, 2002); (2) assisting with school re-entry after hospital stays or extended absences (Shaw & McCabe, 2008); (3) assisting teachers in understanding the child's condition and providing ideas of how to work with the child and his or her parents (DeWalt & Hink, 2009); (4) facilitating positive interactions and relationships between the child and his or her teachers and peers (Freeborn & Mandleco, 2010); and (5) implementing interventions in the classroom that will enhance child coping and academic achievement (Rynard *et al.*, 1998).

COLLABORATING WITH TEACHERS

Mental health professionals should inform teachers of their availability to provide ideas for supporting the child's social and emotional development (Clay *et al.*,

2004). Educating teachers about what to do in an emergency and how to enhance child inclusion in social situations can ease teacher concerns. And, of course, working with the teacher to improve child academic performance can support teachers and child achievement (King *et al.,* 2005). Table **2** presents some references that may be useful for teachers working with children with chronic illnesses in the classroom.

Table 2:   **Resources for Teachers**

Resource	Description
Best *et al.*, (2005). *Teaching Individuals with Physical or Multiple Disabilities: Fifth Edition.*	This text reviews ideas for curriculum adaptation and instructional strategies. Techniques for working with children with physical, neurological, and health problems are reviewed.
McGrath and Johns (2008). *Reaching Students with Diverse Disabilities: Cross-Categorical Ideas and Activities.*	This book provides suggestions for improving children's social and emotional development as well as their language and math skills. The role of specialists and tips for completion of education plans are explained.
Nabors *et al.*, (2009). Ideas for teachers working with children who have medical conditions. M. T. Burton (Ed.). *Special Education in the 21st Century. Series: Education in a Competitive and Globalizing World.* (pp. 155-167). New York: Nova Science Publishers.	This chapter reviews practical ideas to assist teachers in meeting the social emotional and academic needs of children with medical conditions in their classrooms.
Nielsen (2009). *Brief Reference of Student Disabilities…With Strategies for the Classroom: Second Edition.*	This book reviews information about regulations and laws, ideas for creating a positive learning environment, and strategies for educators for several different types of medical conditions.
Phelps (2006). *Chronic health-related disorders in children: Collaborative medical and psychoeducational interventions.*	This book presents ideas for assessment of children's needs for academic accommodations to enrich their learning and inclusion in the classroom.

Helping teachers understand how the child communicates his or her needs can be an invaluable tool in the classroom. For example, some children may not wish to talk much about their illness, while others might like to discuss their condition with peers and the teacher. It may be advisable to set up a meeting with the child, the child's parents, and the child's teacher or teachers in order for them to jointly develop a "care plan" for meeting the child's needs. Allowing the child to become involved in the planning can improve his or her feelings of involvement in care and therefore enhance locus of control for care. If the child is more involved in his or her care, this may, in turn, improve adherence to the medical regimen. The improved communication also can foster a positive relationship between the teacher or teachers and the child, so that the child has a support person that he or she can talk to about having an illness. The open lines of communication and feelings of security can promote asking for help and sharing information, such that adults are able to be more aware of the child's health status and needs. The mental health provider can arrange meetings and then follow-up, checking in with the child's teacher to ensure that medical management is going smoothly in the classroom. If "booster sessions" or additional meetings are needed then the mental health provider can facilitate these sessions, further improving chances for connection between the child and his or her teachers (Nabors *et al.*, 2012).

CHILDREN WITH CANCER

Rynard *et al.,* (1998) presented ideas for assisting children with cancer at school – this illness has good literature to guide best practices in the school setting. Though the focus of their work is on one illness, they addressed issues faced by children with many types of chronic medical conditions. They described several key roles for school-based mental health professionals: (1) helping children cope with absences; (2) teaching children strategies for coping with medical fears; (3) developing emergency medical plans and designing ideas for classroom support for the child; (4) assisting children in coping with side-effects related to medical care; (5) providing counseling and support; (6) consulting and collaborating with parents, school staff, and the medical team; (7) providing interventions to improve academic and cognitive functioning; (8) developing interventions to improve adherence to medical regimens and improving child involvement in self-care; and (9) providing counseling to increase children's coping with emotional and behavioral problems related to living with their illness (see Table **1**). Children with cancer often deal with frequent, long-term absences (Rynard *et al.*, 1998). Helping children make up missed assignments and catch up on lecture material can be critical to their success once they return to school (Worchell-Prevatt *et al.*, 1998). If the child has had a treatment that alters his or her appearance, talking with peers to elicit their help and support and being on-hand to provide supportive counseling to the child him- or herself can ease the transition and improve acceptance of the child. Furthermore, improving the child's relationships or assisting with the development of positive relationships with peers may be a resilience factor for children with cancer (Kim & Yoo, 2009).

SCHOOL REINTEGRATION

School reintegration and readjustment is another area where a mental health provider can assist the child and his or her parents. Prevatt *et al.,* (2000) provide a detailed review of school re-entry programs. Children returning to school often benefit from tutoring, attending school for shortened periods of time, or having a temporary classroom aide to assist them in learning academic concepts they may not have learned prior to their hospitalization or extended absence from school. Shaw and McCabe (2008) developed a reference that provides guidance for school re-entry. They review ideas for hospital-to-school transition for children with chronic illnesses, in light of the changing health care system. Developing care plans or steps for care to administer new medications and manage their side effects is another valuable contribution. New medications, initiated during a hospital stay, can create new problems in adhering to medication schedules and taking medications. The school-based mental health professional can support nursing and other school staff by teaching the child to take an active role in medication management through developing plans to monitor pill taking and developing reward systems for positive actions related to taking new medications (Worchell-Prevatt *et al.*, 1998).

Post-hospitalization, children may feel isolated or different and "set apart" from their classroom peers. The mental health provider can work with the child, through role play, to assist the child in learning how to explain his or her absence and any changes in appearance or medical management that could have resulted from the hospitalization. Moreover, it may be advantageous to identify a peer who can be a "buddy" to support the child in entering group interactions and reintegrating into social networks in the classroom (Sexson & Madan-Swain, 1995). If a child is physically limited, such as being wheelchair –bound, the mental health provider can work with the child's teacher and other school staff to modify the environment. For example, if the child is weak or physically limited, one idea would be to improve the physical layout of recreational spaces, such as playgrounds, so that the child can more easily join in play and ongoing interactions (Nabors *et al.*, 2007).

Many children who have chronic illnesses do not want to "stand out" or appear to be different from their peers who do not have chronic health conditions. Determining the child's needs for privacy and confidentiality regarding his or her medical condition, and educating school staff about the child's preferences, will help adults to meet the child where he or she is and to create an environment where the child feels secure and confident. Consequently, steps and directions from care plans need to be implemented in a manner that promotes the best possible inclusion of the child with the illness, so that he or she receives as much integration into the normal school setting and routine as possible. Many of the children who have chronic illnesses would like to "blend in" and "fly under the radar," and in other words cope with their condition without it being too noticeable by peers. Though this may not be completely possible, involving the child in care planning is a way to learn if the child needs to be "unobtrusive" in terms of his or her medical management in the classroom and other settings, such as during recess or lunch.

CASE STUDIES

Case Study 1: Girl with Cystic Fibrosis

Consider the case of Ella, a young girl with Cystic Fibrosis, who has missed a significant amount of school related to having a severe case of pneumonia. Ella is in 2nd grade and is shy. She often has had to leave the classroom for percussion therapy to clear mucous from her lungs – related to her Cystic Fibrosis. Also, because of her condition, she must eat a very high calorie diet, which has brought her undue peer attention. Other children have asked her why she is "so skinny" when she eats "two lunches every lunch period." Ella has also faced some peer teasing because she is thin, with one little boy, nicknaming her "the twig," which became known to and used by other children who were members of her class.

Ella's teacher is strict and has difficulty coping with changes to the classroom routine. Thus, Ella's absences and those times she leaves for percussion therapy are considered "interruptions" that "disrupt class routine and progress" by the teacher. Ella's teacher is somewhat resistant to developing and explaining make-up assignments when children miss class, and Ella has missed quite a lot of time related to her pneumonia and resultant hospital stay. She reports fear related to returning to school. Her mother contacted the school psychologist, a mental health provider who has been working with Ella since she began kindergarten at her elementary school.

After a phone conversation, the school psychologist and Ella's mother met to develop a plan for helping Ella catch up on her school work, improving relationships with others in her classroom, and assisting her in coping with her diet and therapy sessions that made her "stand out" from her peers. This plan also involved ideas for explaining Ella's condition to her teacher and involving the school nurse in sessions to explain Ella's condition to children in the class. The plan is outlined in Table **3**.

Table 3: **Outline of School Care Plan for Ella**

Teacher	School Nurse	Mental Health Provider
School-home note delivered through email with daily class work and homework assignments.	Provide information about condition to class.	Provide information about needs in the classroom and connect teacher with medical information.
Respond to child requests; improve flexibility with absences from class.	Have medications available; back-up plan for administration of medications if nurse is absent; convey information from the medical team.	Monitor social-emotional functioning; assign peer buddy; observe and informally assess peer acceptance.
Learn ways to support child adherence to medical appointments and care.	Provide input and assist in development of school plan.	Develop plans to provide physical therapy at school to reduce time outside the classroom.
Assist child in completing class work and homework; provide make-up work.	Convey information on medical management and what to do in case of emergency to others at school.	Check for missed assignments; assist in locating tutors.
		Weekly counseling to support Ella in re-adjustment to school; connect with parents to update them about Ella's progress and provide parent counseling as needed.

As shown in Table **3**, the teacher can play a key role in assisting Ella's academic progress by supporting her learning needs when she is absent from the classroom.

It also will be important for the teacher to be accepting of Ella's needs to miss class for therapy appointments and other medical appointments. The teacher should update Ella's parents on her academic progress with a school-home note, sent weekly. The teacher also can support peer tutoring efforts to assist Ella in "catching up" when she is completing missed assignments.

The school nurse can provide education about Ella's medical condition to the teacher and other children in the classroom. A class meeting can be a time to educate peers about Ella's condition and ways to help her in the classroom and on the playground. The school nurse can also be a liaison with the medical team to learn about changes to medical care and ways to best assist Ella when she returns to school after hospitalizations. The school nurse also may need to connect with the physical education teacher and teachers for other special classes, such as art and music, so that these teachers are made aware of any special planning for Ella.

The mental health professional or provider can provide counseling for Ella, to support her in coping with school re-integration and with dealing with any feelings related to her previous emergency hospitalization to recover from pneumonia. Communicating with parents and offering supportive counseling is a key component of comprehensive care planning for Ella. The mental health professional can assign a school buddy to help Ella complete missed assignments. The school counselor also could meet with the teacher to explain Ella's emotional functioning and together they can brainstorm to develop interventions to increase her social involvement on the playground and during other "special" classes, such as art class. If any field trips are planned, the mental health provider can serve as a liaison, connecting the teacher to the child's medical team and Ella's parents, in order to develop any special planning to ensure Ella's success on the field trip. The mental health provider also can hold a group session to explain Ella's medical condition and provide ideas for ways her peers can help Ella – for example – waiting for her if she falls behind on the playground or helping her carry her books if they are too heavy for her. The mental health provider also can be a support for Ella, helping her find out about missed assignments and developing planning with her teacher to set a timeline for catching up on the work she missed while in the hospital.

Case Study 2: Boy with Type 1 Diabetes

This case study begins with a review of a study examining "needs at school" for young children with diabetes. Children's opinions were assessed at a diabetes camp, during a medical education period. Children responded to a survey assessing their needs for support during the past school year (Nabors *et al.*, 2003). Most of those youth surveyed, reported that they did feel supported in their diabetes care while at school. Some did state that they required more assistance from their teacher in helping them recognize hypoglycemic episodes, which were difficult for them to detect. During these episodes the child needed teacher support to test blood sugar on an immediate basis. If the child had to go to see the nurse, they preferred to walk with another friend who was in the class. Children also reported benefitting when teachers communicated with parents about snacks that needed to be on hand when they felt "low." One barrier to good management occurred when teachers were not supportive of the child's needs to test blood sugars regularly and when thinking he or she might be "high" or "low." Some children did not want to test in front of peers and classroom rules for remaining in the classroom made it challenging for the child to have privacy when testing blood sugar levels. Some children also reported experiencing teasing at school or limited selections of foods that were appropriate for them to eat if they had to "buy" lunch. With this brief review of the children's perceptions in mind, we will consider the case of Daniel, a 13-year-old with diabetes who was struggling to maintain lower blood sugar levels and improve disease management.

Daniel requested a visit with the school mental health counselor, because he was upset about his diabetes management in the classroom. Upon meeting Daniel it was noted that he appeared mild-mannered and was well-dressed and groomed. This presentation varied with his teacher's characterization of Daniel as a child who could be unruly and act in an unpredictable manner, especially toward the end of the school day. Upon meeting the counselor, Daniel immediately explained that he was often "going low" at the end of the school day. He discussed his typical low behaviors as being "disorganized, grumpy, and 'out of it' so that paying attention is very difficult." Daniel reported that he was low, because he did not have snacks available in the classroom, which would be very important to him, because he had a first-bell, early lunch period. The reason he did not have snacks available is his teacher, Ms. McMann, had a no food policy in her room.

Daniel provided the school counselor with his parents' home telephone number during this impromptu session and the counselor contacted his parents to determine if Daniel could participate in regular counseling. Similar to her son, his mother was very concerned about the teacher's lack of understanding of his disease management and the importance of having snacks to address "lows" (hyperglycemic episodes) available in the classroom.

The school counselor first requested to speak with Daniel's classroom teacher during her class planning period. They met within two days and discussed Daniel's fears related to having a hyperglycemic episode in the classroom. They talked about his need for privacy when testing his blood sugar. Moreover, they discussed how snacks could be used to treat low blood sugars. At the end of their conversation the teacher agreed to meet with Daniel's mother as well as the school district nurse, who was also a diabetes educator. The meeting with the diabetes educator would be to provide the teacher with information about diabetes, dietary needs of the child, and symptoms of low and high blood sugars in children with diabetes.

The nurse from the diabetes team provided a written report, detailing some key ideas for management of Daniel's low and high episodes and ideas for helping him test his blood sugars in a confidential setting. The teacher also requested ideas for emergency contacts and emergency planning. The teacher and school-based counselor shared this information from the medical team at a parent meeting with Daniel's mother. His mother provided ideas for snacks that were especially helpful when Daniel experienced a "low." Drinking lots of water, where other children could not see him, was a request for handling high blood glucose levels. When supplied with information from the medical team, the teacher was much more confident and receptive to meeting with and sharing information with Daniel's mother. The mental health counselor served as a recorder and she took notes during their conversation, which she then shared with the medical team and school nurse. At this point, the nurse on the medical team recommended that there be a team meeting, consisting of the school nurse, school-based mental health provider, and Daniel's mother and teacher to develop a care plan for Daniel.

At the meeting, which occurred in Daniel's classroom, the group worked together to develop a care plan to maximize Daniel's diabetes management while at school. His care plan included emergency contact information, a section on his needs for testing his blood sugar, and a section on steps for care when he was experiencing either a "high" or a "low." Luckily the nurse was on site every day, so the teacher agreed to send Daniel to the nurse, with a peer as a "buddy" when he reported feeling high or low. She also agreed to keep a can of soda on hand in the classroom and glucose tablets to help Daniel treat hyperglycemic episodes or "lows" that occurred in the classroom. The teacher agreed to contact Daniel's mother weekly, *via* telephone, to share information about Daniel's diabetes management. Finally, the teacher agreed to allow Daniel to step outside the classroom door to test blood glucose levels, in order for him to feel less self-conscious around his classmates. It was agreed that Daniel's teacher would meet, accompanied by the school counselor, to share results of the planning meeting with Daniel. Daniel's attitude toward his teacher began to change, and in the long run he had fewer missed assignments and began to perform better on tests. These actions resulted in further improvement in the teacher-student relationship.

Daniel had reported that the cafeteria remained a difficult setting for his diabetes management. A meeting between the cook at the cafeteria and Daniel's mother was arranged. They developed ideas for modifying the school lunch to include more vegetables and protein, which greatly helped Daniel. To do this, the cook made some lunches available with more vegetables and protein. To her surprise, some other children requested these lunch options and the healthy lunch option became a staple in the school cafeteria during lunch.

This case study exemplified the "connecting" role that the mental health counselor can play in getting "key players" such as teachers and parents to meet to determine care plans. In addition, the mental health counselor's efforts lead to improved academic achievement for Daniel and improved healthy food options for lunch for those peers who were interested in and requested the "healthy lunch" option. A summary of modifications developed to improve school-based diabetes management for Daniel is presented in Table **4**.

Table 4:   Outline of School Care Plan for Daniel

Teacher	School Staff: Nurse and Cook	Mental Health Provider
School-home note delivered through email on a weekly basis; open communication with parent(s), with a problem-solving orientation.

Improve flexibility related to blood glucose testing.

Have snacks available in class.

Assign a peer "buddy" to walk with Daniel to the nurse if he was feeling "high" or "low".

Learn ways to support child adherence to blood glucose testing regimen.

Assist child in completing class work and homework. | **Nurse**: have snacks on hand. Communicate with medical team and develop emergency medical planning. Have insulin available in nurses office; back-up plan for administration of medications if nurse is absent; convey information from the medical team.

Cook: Modify lunch plan so that healthy choices to facilitate Daniel's diabetes management are available so that he could buy lunch at school – just like his friends! Adding healthier options can lead to positive change for other children. | Arrange meetings to develop a care plan and to facilitate school-home communication.

Provide information about needs in the classroom and connect teacher with the parent.

Support Daniel as he deals with emotions related to his relationship with his teacher and difficulties with classroom diabetes management; counseling sessions as needed.

Monitor social-emotional functioning; assist teacher in planning for a buddy system to walk Daniel to the nurse if he was experiencing a "high" or "low"; observe and informally assess peer acceptance.

Check for missed assignments; long-term contact to ensure maintenance of care plan. |

As a result of the case management role, and the key connections, Daniel's context improved and his relationship with the teacher and school connectedness subsequently improved. This resulted in improved confidence for diabetes management on the part of Daniel's teacher and for Daniel himself. Although sessions with Daniel became less frequent, the school counselor continued to "check in" with brief meetings with Daniel and his teacher to ensure that his diabetes management and school achievement remained "on track."

Case Study 3: Girl with Vision Problems

This case describes Laura, a 3 year-old girl with amblyopia or a lazy eye. She wore very thick glasses and an eye patch for some of the school day. Laura attended a daycare that her parents called "preschool" while they went to work each day. The eye patch was to help straighten her lazy eye, which was her right eye that tended to bend to the left and was not "looking straight ahead and centered" like her left eye. The other children did not understand her eye patch and called her "pirate face" and kept asking her where her ship was. Laura was a very sensitive little girl and the teasing often hurt her feelings. She was too shy and quiet to tell the teacher and most of the teasing typically occurred on the playground. The eye patch did not fix Laura's eye and she had to go to the children's hospital to have a surgery to correct her eye muscles, which were causing her lazy eye. After her surgery, which went very well, Laura stayed home for a few days to recover. Her right eye, however, was very red and Laura still had to wear a patch at school. One child in her classroom began calling Laura "red eye," and "ugly eye" which made Laura cry.

The name-calling occurred for 3 days. On the fourth day Laura refused to go to school. She cried and said that she would rather be at the hospital where, "everyone was nice about my eye and patch." On day 5, Laura again cried and tried to stay home from school. This time when her mother asked Laura what was wrong, she began talking about the boy who called her "eye names" and made the other children laugh on the playground. Laura's mother asked if the teacher knew about the name-calling. Laura said that she had never told the teacher about being called "pirate" or "ugly eye."

Laura's mother called the counselor, a specialist in child health or pediatric psychology. The counselor scheduled an appointment with Laura's mother to learn more about the situation and then talked with Laura's teacher by telephone. After this, the counselor met with Laura and her mother. She got to know Laura for a few minutes and then brought out some dolls. The counselor and Laura drew a playground and then Laura took some of the dolls and re-enacted her perceptions of her own playground experience. Laura held one doll she called "Lizzy." She talked about how Lizzy had an ugly eye that other kids talked about. Then, she held a boy doll and told a story about how the boy called Lizzy "red eye, pirate, and ugly eye." She showed how the other little girls (dolls she held) became afraid and would not play with Lizzie. Lizzie really wanted to be at school and wanted the other children to understand that she had a surgery and needed a little bit of time for her eye to "get well and be straight." At the end of the session, all the dolls were friends and understood about Lizzy's eye and that it would heal soon.

After the play, the counselor spoke again with Laura's mother. They decided that Laura's mother would call the teacher and see if Laura's counselor could come to the classroom and explain Laura's medical condition, surgery, and the recovery process. The teacher and daycare director agreed that the counselor could come to the school and talk with the children in Laura's class. The counselor came to circle time later the same week. During circle time the counselor told a story through doll play. The story in her pretend play was about "Annie," a little girl with a lazy eye that was not looking straight ahead. The counselor put an eye patch on the doll (Annie). The counselor stated, "Annie wore an eye patch on her strong eye for a while to help make her other eye work hard so it could become straighter." She showed all the other dolls playing with Annie and having lots of fun with her.

A little girl raised her hand and asked if Annie's eye would get better. The counselor replied, "Yes, I think it will." Next, the little girl asked if the girl in the "play" was Laura. The counselor said "Yes, Annie is like Laura. She wants to come to school like Laura, she is just like all of the other children, she just has to wear an eye patch to help her eye heal and become straight." After this, the little girl asked if Laura could play and run like the other children at recess. The counselor said Laura could do so, and would really like to play with the other children.

The next day, Laura went to school with her mother and they met the counselor at the director's office. Then the group went to Laura's classroom. The teacher warmly greeted Laura, her mother and the counselor. Then, the teacher announced to the children, "The counselor is here to talk with you again. Laura is here too and so is her mother. Let's all say 'hello' to all of them." The children then greeted Laura and her mother. Then, the teacher said, "Yesterday we talked about a little girl who had an eye surgery and had a red eye, but came back to school. She also wore an eye patch. This is just like Laura." The children asked Laura some questions about her eye patch, which she and her counselor answered. After this, Laura's mother left and she was able to stay with her class and have a successful playground experience.

During the following weeks, the teacher continued to redirect and model appropriate friendship on the playground for the boy who had teased Laura. The other children, especially three of the girls, played with Laura every day. Laura began to report "I like school." She had one of the three little girls who played with her on the playground over to her home for a successful play date. The teacher sent weekly reports to Laura's mother, letting her know that all was well in the classroom. Laura continued to have a successful preschool year and she no longer needed to see the counselor.

CONCLUSION

Children with medical conditions can benefit from a supportive and flexible educational environment. This can be achieved through care plans that provide ideas for helping the child complete missed school work. These plans can outline emergency planning and require regular communication and "updates" between the teacher and the child's parents or caregivers. Obtaining updates from the child's medical team after hospitalization is critical. If needed, the mental health clinician can provide therapy and support to ease school re-integration or assist the child in coping with any depression or anxiety related to school absences and completion of school work. The mental health professional or school nurse can explain the child's medical condition to teachers and peers, thereby improving understanding and acceptance.

Care plans have the potential to inform teachers and staff about each child's needs so that they can respond appropriately. The school mental health professional can assist with developing care plans, assessing child cognitive, social, and emotional functioning, and evaluating child participation and adjustment in the school setting. The school mental health professional may serve as a case manager, involving the child, parent, medical team and other school staff in developing and implementing the care plan.

ACKNOWLEDGEMENTS

None declared.

CONFLICT OF INTEREST

The author confirms that this chapter contents have no conflict of interest.

REFERENCES

American Academy of Pediatrics Council on School Health (2009) Policy Statement-Guidance for the administration of medication in school. *Pediatrics, 124*(4), 1244-1251.

American Diabetes Association (2004). Co-Sponsor: Disability Rights Education & Defense Fund. *Sample Section 504 Plan*. Retrieved on February 21, 2011 from http://www.ibsgroup.org/chronickids/504.pdf.

Best, S. J., Wolff-Heller, K., & Bigge, J. L. (2005). *Teaching Individuals with Physical or Multiple Disabilities: Fifth Edition*. Upper Saddle River, NJ: Pearson: Merrill Prentice Hall.

Clay, D., Cortina, S., Harper, D., Cocco, K., & Drotar, D. (2004). Schoolteachers' experiences with childhood chronic illness. *Children's Health Care, 33*(3), 227-239.

DeWalt, D. A., & Hink, A. (2009). Health literacy and child health outcomes: A systematic review of the literature. *Pediatrics, 124*, S265-S274.

Forrest, C. B., Simpson, L., & Clancy, C. (1997). Child health services research: Challenges and opportunities. *Journal of the American Medical Association, 277*(22), 1787–1793.

Freeborn, D., & Mandleco, B. (2010). Childhood educational experiences of women with cerebral palsy. *Journal of School Nursing, 26*(4), 310-319.

Kim, D. H., & Yoo, I. Y. (2009). Factors associated with resilience of school age children with cancer. *Journal of Paediatrics and Child Health, 46*, 431-436.

King, A.A., Tang, S., Ferguson, K.L., & DeBaun, M.R. (2005). An education program to increase teacher knowledge about sickle cell disease. *Journal of School Health, 75*(1), 11-14.

Jaff, J. C. (2010). *Know your rights: A handbook for patients with chronic illness*. Farmington, CT: Advocacy for Patients with Chronic Illness.

McGrath, M. Z., & Johns, B. H. (2008). *Reaching students with diverse disabilities: Cross categorical ideas and activities*. Lanham, MD: Rowman & Littlefield Education.

Nabors, L. A., McGrady, M. E., Rosenzweig, K. J., & Srivorakiat, L. (2007). Improving the competence of preschoolers with disabilities on playgrounds. *Early Childhood Services, 4*, 235-247.

Nabors, L., Olsen, B., & Henderson, E. (2009). Ideas for teachers working with children who have medical conditions. M. T. Burton (Ed.). *Special Education in the 21st Century. Series: Education in a Competitive and Globalizing World*. (pp. 155-167). New York: Nova Science Publishers.

Nabors, L., Ritchey, P. N., Sebera, K., & Ludke, R. L. (2012). Mental health providers and children with medical conditions in school. In M. Haines and A. Pearce (Eds.). *Child and School Psychology* (pp. 85-106). New York: Nova Science Publishers.

Nielsen, L. B. (2009). *Brief reference of student disabilities…with strategies for the classroom.* Thousand Oaks, CA: Corwin Press: Sage.

Nolan, K. W., Orlando, M., & Liptak, G. S. (2007). Care coordination services for children with special health care needs: Are we family-centered yet? *Families, Systems, & Health, 25*(3), 293-306.

Peebles-Wilkins, W. (2006). Editorial: Responding to children with chronic illness. *Children & Schools, 28*, 67-68.

Phelps, L. (Ed.) (2006). *Chronic health-related disorders in children: Collaborative medical and psychoeducational interventions.* Washington DC: American Psychological Association.

Prevatt, F. F., Heffer, R. W., & Lowe, P. A. (2000). A review of school reintegration programs for children with cancer. *Journal of School Psychology, 38*, 447-467.

Rynard, D. W., Chambers, A., Klinck, A. M., & Gray, J. D. (1998). School support programs for chronically ill children: Evaluating adjustment of children with cancer at school. *Children's Health Care, 27*, 31-46.

Sexson, S., & Madan-Swain, A. (1995). The chronically ill child in school. *School Psychology Quarterly, 10*, 359-368.

Shaw, S., & McCabe, P. (2008). Hospital-to-school transition for children with chronic illness: Meeting the new challenges of an evolving health care system. *Psychology in the Schools, 45* (1), 74-87.

Smith, F. J., Taylor, K. M. G., Newbould, J., & Keady, S. (2008). Medicines for chronic illness at school: Experiences and concerns of young people and their parents. *Journal of Clinical Pharmacy and Therapeutics, 33*(5), 537-544.

Vance, Y. H., & Eiser, C. (2002). The school experience of the child with cancer. *Child: Care, Health, and Development, 28*, 5-19.

Worchel-Prevatt, F. F., Heffer, R. W., Prevatt, B. C., Miner, J., Young-Saleme, T., Horgan, D., Lopez, M., Rae, W. A., & Frankel, L. (1998). A school reentry program for chronically ill children. *Journal of School Psychology, 36*, 261-279.

CHAPTER 5

Assessment of Children's School Functioning

Laura A. Nabors[*]

Health Education Program, School of Human Services, University of Cincinnati, 468 Dyer Hall, Mail Location 0068, Cincinnati, Ohio, OH 45221-0068, USA

Abstract: This chapter reviews ideas for assessment of children's school functioning and adds information about written care plans in the school setting, which are termed Individual Education Plans and Section 504 plans in the United States. Literature on school planning for children with special health care needs is reviewed and roles of the school psychologist are outlined. Resources for special education teams, to enhance knowledge about child chronic medical conditions, are presented.

Keywords: Academic skills, assessment, educational planning, school behaviors, school functioning, school psychologist.

INTRODUCTION

Regular assessment of children's functioning, particularly cognitive skills, is indicated for many children with chronic illnesses or developmental disabilities (Irwin & Elam, 2011). If necessary, the child should receive an Individual Education Plan (IEP) to ensure that he or she has opportunities to have his or her educational needs met in the least restrictive setting. Some children with medical conditions may experience deficits in cognitive functioning related to their condition (Individuals with Disabilities Education Act, 2004). Others may experience behavioral or emotional problems that are detrimental to their functioning at school. Some children may experience sensory issues or have difficulties with the development of speech and language skills. In a report in the *Future of Children*, researchers documented that over 5.5 million children face activity restrictions, which significantly change many children's school involvement and experiences (Halfon *et al.*, 2012). These researchers noted that

*Address correspondence to Laura A. Nabors: Health Education Program, School of Human Services, University of Cincinnati, 468 Dyer Hall, Mail Location 0068, Cincinnati, Ohio, OH 45221-0068, USA; Tel: 513-556-5537; Fax: 513-556-3898; E-mail: naborsla@ucmail.uc.edu

having a chronic condition can be a heavier burden, even in terms of school functioning, for children who are residing in poverty, and thus special efforts to ensure these children's academic success may be warranted.

After an initial assessment of the child's abilities is completed, then yearly updates or perhaps quarterly updates may be needed to examine for change in child functioning (Individuals with Disabilities Education Act, 2004). At update or interim meetings a full evaluation may not be required. A team meeting with a member of the child's special education team, a counselor, the child's parent, and some type of contact (*via* email, written letter, or telephone) may be sufficient to update current educational planning needs. After three years, however, the child should receive a re-evaluation of his or her cognitive, achievement, and psychosocial (especially behavioral and emotional) functioning. This may ensure that the child's educational planning is accurate and shifts to meet changes in the child as he or she passes through different developmental phases or copes with illness-related issues that could possibly impact his or her personal functioning and school performance. Additionally, when the child enters high school, regular meetings to examine academic progress and emotional functioning should also include discussion of future plans for the transition to adulthood.

For the "Project School Pathways Project" a screening instrument was used to determine the school needs of 1,457 children in the fourth through sixth grades (Forrest *et al.*, 2011). Children and their caregivers resided in Maryland and Virginia in the United States (U. S.). Results indicated that 33% of the youth had a special health care need. In order to meet the needs of these youth, collaboration with health care professionals assisted in ensuring their well-being. Forrest *et al.*, (2011) recommended that research will be needed to determine long-term outcomes of children with chronic conditions and their long-term educational needs. They found that children with special health care needs may experience cognitive sequelae related to complications from their illnesses.

In some cases, specialists outside the school setting are needed to evaluate children with certain types of conditions. For example, children with conditions that impact neurologic functioning may need special evaluations, by experts on their medical team or at local children's hospitals to determine interventions to meet their involved and unique educational needs in the school setting (Armstrong 2012; Bitsko *et al.*, 2009). Moreover, children with conditions such as: autism, mental retardation, blindness, and sensory deficits may need specialists to provide recommendations to optimize their educational opportunities at school (Boulet *et al.*, 2009). Special screenings to determine needs for medical equipment and therapies may be another avenue for ensuring appropriate academic modifications for young children with special health care needs (Bitsko *et al.*, 2009; Gargiulo & Kilgo, 2012).

Because they face so many challenges and worry about their longevity, children with chronic illnesses also may not always see value, in terms of "long-term" gain, in participating in school and working hard on academic pursuits. A lack of involvement in social interactions can also have negative effects on social growth and friendships, thereby negatively impacting social development. As such, counseling and mental health services delivered in the school setting may be warranted to help children cope with anxiety and, at times, difficulties they may have in terms of performing to the best of their abilities in the school setting.

As mentioned, children with chronic illness are at risk for lower academic achievement (Forrest *et al.*, 2011; Suris *et al.,* 2004). Frequent or bi-yearly assessment to determine level of cognitive functioning and achievement in different academic skill areas may be warranted to ensure that the child has the potential to meet academic demands associated with his or her grade level. Children with chronic illnesses may experience bullying, which further disenfranchises them, in terms of school involvement (Forrest *et al.*, 2011). Additionally, if a child has significant emotional and behavioral concerns, in addition to chronic health problems, the child may face elevated risk for school problems and low academic achievement. Forrest *et al.,* (2011) noted that the multiple "risk" indices for children with chronic medical conditions suggested a need to identify their school needs and intervene early, in order to ensure a positive academic trajectory and school success for these children.

Halfon *et al.,* (2012) suggested that how an individual with a special health condition copes within his or her environment can shed light on the modifications required for him or her to be successful. They recommended using the World

Health Organization's International Classification of Functioning, Disability, and Health's definition of disabilities or special needs to guide understanding of helping individuals to fully participate in their environments (World Health Organization: International Classification of Functioning, 2001 as cited in Halfon *et al.*, 2012). When using this definition as a starting point, professionals who are developing special education plans have a comprehensive conceptualization of child functioning that considers social, emotional, cognitive and academic functioning. Halfon *et al.*, (2012) recommended looking at the fit of the child in his or her environment and a perspective of making modifications to move toward the fullest inclusion possible, making modifications so that the child can participate in the school setting to the best of his or her academic, social, and developmental abilities. This broad, inclusive conceptualization may set an orientation that is pro-child and pro-positive school environment that can maximize the child's chances of being included and performing well at school.

SECTION 504 PLAN IN THE UNITED STATES

A child who does not qualify for an IEP based on delays in his or functioning may benefit from receiving a section 504 plan for having another type of health impairment (U.S. Department of Education, 2007). A Section 504 plan allows a child to have accommodations based on his or her medical and mental health needs so that he or she can achieve to the best of his or her ability in the school setting. This is a written plan for those with "other health impairments," such as chronic illness, so that their educational needs can be met in the least restrictive environment to promote their academic potential. For instance, a child who has Type 1 Diabetes, but is not experiencing any behavioral or emotional problems or any problems with academic achievement might benefit from having a 504 plan in order to facilitate diabetes management. The Section 504 medical plan for optimal involvement in school should be evaluated on a regular basis. There could be a written plan for what to do if a child experiences hyperglycemic or hypoglycemic episodes in the school setting. Snacks that the child prefers to treat a "low" could be specified so that the teacher and school nurse know what types of "low snacks" to have on hand. Similarly, a child with asthma might benefit from a 504 plan to document what to do on case of an asthma attack and to document, in writing, that the child needs to have his or her inhaler with him or herself at all times during the school day. A good resource for mental health practitioners and others on the special education team working with children with chronic illnesses in schools was developed by Daniel Clay (2004), and is entitled, "Helping school children with chronic health conditions: A practical guide." This book has ideas that can help shape the development of optimal 504 planning and classroom assistance for children with chronic health conditions[1].

Madaus and Shaw (2004) described how a Section 504 plan works as well as differences in the plan when one compares Subpart D and Subpart E. Section 504 is part of the Rehabilitation Act of 1973 and addresses civil rights. The goal is for a student with physical and mental impairments to receive the accommodations needed for him or her to receive an appropriate educational experience. It is noteworthy that physical and mental limitations must be significant, in that either one causes a limitation in a major life function. The Section 504 plan differs when one considers secondary *versus* post-secondary education. The first part, Subpart D, addresses educational systems that receive federal assistance at the secondary level. Schools or educational institutions that receive federal assistance must offer educational opportunities that help to "level the playing field" in terms of assisting a child with a physical or mental impairment to achieve to the best of his or her abilities. The schools must provide an evaluation or go through an evaluation process to ensure that the student receives appropriate accommodations so that he or she can be successful in reaching his or her academic potential and in learning at school. Some schools are very willing to develop section 504 plans for children with chronic illnesses. Alternately, due to paperwork required in setting up special plans, other school special education teams may prefer to make changes to the child's learning plan in the classroom without implementing a 504 plan. It may be advisable to request the 504 plan, as it ensures that changes are made.

In Subpart E, which addresses the post-secondary level, the goals are similar. However, the college or post-secondary institution (such as a vocational school) sets the requirements for entrance standards (Madaus & Shaw, 2004). Then, once

---

[1]Clay's work is discussed in Nabors, L., Akin-Little, A., Little, S., & Iobst, E. (2008). Teachers' knowledge about chronic illnesses. For the mini-series: Psychology's contribution to education: Improving educational opportunities for all children. *Psychology in the Schools, 45*, 217-226.

the student meets the admission requirements and enters the program, it is the institution's responsibility to provide opportunities and accommodate the student's learning needs so that he or she has equal opportunities to complete school and perform to the best of his or her academic abilities. For Subpart E, an evaluation is not required. It may be the student's responsibility to provide documentation so that special accommodations can be made to facilitate his or her learning in the post-secondary environment.

It is important to remember that IEP paperwork and Section 504 paperwork do not necessarily automatically follow a student to the post-secondary level. Adler *et al.,* (2008) reported that planning for college and adult years is an important part of educational support for children with chronic medical conditions as these children may have limited success in the college environment as they attempt to cope with their illnesses. Educators need information to understand their special needs, so that their college performance is accelerated.

A Section 504 plan could also have requirements for regular evaluation of the child's cognitive functioning, which is important for many children who have chronic illness, as there is evidence for cognitive changes associated with many types of chronic illnesses (Irwin & Elam, 2011). Suris *et al.,* (2004) also highlighted the notion that cognitive functioning should be assessed on a regular basis for children with many types of chronic conditions. Specifically, they pointed to diabetes, with cognitive change related to prolonged and repeated episodes of hypoglycemia, and change in cognitive ability for children with sickle cell anemia due to cerebrovascular incidents may impact school performance and long-term achievement in the school setting. Moreover, it may be advisable to involve the child's medical team in the development of the plan. The school staff and a representative of the child's medical team may need to meet regularly to ensure that communication is maintained (Adler *et al.*, 2008). The health care system has been evolving as technology has been linked to improved medical care and medical interventions are continually evolving and improving. Thus, continued updates from the medical team can provide a window of best management of specific medical conditions. Moreover, the medical team should be contacted when the child faces any type of serious hospitalization in order to ensure a smooth hospital-to-school transition for the child with a chronic illness (Shaw & McCabe, 2008).

Planning for make-up work due to medically-related school absences also can be recorded in the 504 Plan (U.S. Department of Education, 2007). For example, a child with arthritis may need an extra set of textbooks to keep at home, because all of the books he or she would need to bring home in order to do homework, would be too heavy to carry, and might aggravate arthritis-related pain. Planning for make-up work and "keeping up with the class" may be especially important from some children, as frequent school absences due to a flare-up of disease conditions or multiple medical visits may be problematic. Planning for social experiences and checking social involvement of the child with a chronic medical condition also may be important, because when these children miss a lot of school they can feel "left out" of normal social interactions and the development of peer relationships that occur when a child is able to attend school on a regular basis (Irwin & Elam, 2011).

Absences are common for all types of illnesses, including those that involve the experience of chronic pain. Logan *et al*., (2008) examined school impairment in adolescents between the ages of 12 through 17 years who were experiencing chronic pain. They collected information from adolescents, parents, school records and teachers. The reason for their study was a concern that youth experiencing chronic pain can experience increased absences and impaired school functioning. Their results indicated that approximately 44% of parents reported that adolescents' grades had dropped since they began to experience chronic pain. The most common report was that grades were down one level (or letter grade). Pain duration and intensity and gender were not related to school performance for youth experiencing chronic pain.

Interestingly, parent and adolescent report were consistent with school records, suggesting that clinicians can get an accurate view of how things are going at school by asking either the adolescent or parent about school functioning (Logan *et al*., 2008). Although teacher data was difficult to obtain, it was determined that teachers perceived children with chronic pain to be well-adjusted. Some of the common adjustments made to help youth when experiencing pain were to send the student to the nurse, send the student home, or grant extensions on assignments. The groups with the highest number of school absences were children with functional abdominal pain and "non-migraine" pain compared to children classified in other pain groups, such as those with neuropathic pain or migraine pain.

ROLE OF THE CHILD OR SCHOOL PSYCHOLOGIST

Regular assessment of the child's cognitive and achievement skills (either yearly or bi-yearly) may be indicated if the child's chronic condition is one that impacts his or her cognitive functioning. In addition to cognitive and achievement levels, the school psychologist or child psychologist may need to conduct a regular assessment of the child's emotional and behavioral functioning. Similarly, a school counselor who works with the child to address mental health concerns may provide an update about the child's progress and changes in functioning as well as ideas for future goals to improve psychosocial development. If the school does not have the specialized assessment tools, then referral to a local children's hospital or a University Affiliated Program with specialists in the assessment of special health care needs may be the optimal way to access measurement tools and expertise to develop the most inclusive school plan for the child.

Referral to child psychiatrists and developmental pediatricians may provide key data to optimize mental, physical and emotional development. They also may update planning for medication management. Moreover, the school or child psychologist may benefit from having an index of private or hospital-based speech and language, physical therapy, and occupational therapy experts to refer children to in order for them to receive the specialized evaluations needed to ensure the most expertise in developing recommendations to enhance their functioning and academic performance.

Another common activity for a school-based psychologist in the United States is to assess child functioning for triennial or three-year evaluations to update Individual Education Plans. At a minimum, these evaluations involve administrations of a test of cognitive functioning and school achievement skills as well as an evaluation of child adaptive functioning at school and at home (when indicated). Liaison work with the school staff and the medical team is a component of best-practice, in order to update members in each group about the child's progress and functioning. In cases where cognitive delays are significant enough to warrant a diagnosis of mental retardation or significant developmental delay in cognitive functioning, then the psychologist also needs access to measures designed to evaluate adaptive functioning so that appropriate educational planning can be implemented. Table **1** presents important resources for special education teams and school psychologists.

Table 1:   Resources for Providing Services in Schools

Armstrong, T. (2012). *Neurodiversity in the classroom: Strength-based strategies to help students with special needs succeed in school and life*. Alexandria, VA: ASCD Publishers.
Barraclough, C., & Machek, G. (2010). School psychologists' role concerning children with chronic illnesses in schools. *Journal of Applied School Psychology, 26*(2), 132-148.
Clay, D. L. (2004). *Helping schoolchildren with chronic health conditions: A practical guide*. The Guilford Practical Intervention in School Series. New York: Guilford Press.
Gargiulo, R., & Kilgo, J. L. (2012). *An Introduction to Young Children with Special Needs: Birth Through Age Eight: Fourth Edition*. Cengage Learning.
Guilford, R., & Upton, G. (2006). *Special Educational Needs*. New York: Routledge.
Power, T. J., & Bradley-Klug, K. L. (2013). *Pediatric school psychology: Conceptualization, applications, and strategies for leadership development. In the school-based practice in action series*. New York: Routledge.

Another important role in the care of a young child with chronic illness may be service coordination. The school psychologist may be in a good position to fulfill the role as a case manager. Child specialists in social work may serve as case managers to organize service delivery and coordination for the child. Coordination of the many appointments and specialty services through the school can be especially helpful for parents residing in low-income families who do not have the transportation to get a child to multiple medical appointments. The case manager can schedule service delivery at the school and serve as a central person to organize the specialized assessments and services that the child needs to ensure a positive developmental trajectory (Bitsko *et al.*, 2009; Boulet *et al.*, 2009; Garguilo & Kilgo, 2012). The next section of this chapter presents information associated with school-based evaluation of children with two different types of medical conditions.

CASE STUDIES

Case Study 1: Girl with HIV

Kenya is a seven-year-old girl, who is Latina, and has HIV/AIDS. Her mother has not yet told her of her HIV status, in order to protect her from stigmatized reactions from peers. Her mother's philosophy has been "do not tell and pretend it is not there." Kenya has a lot of questions about her many doctors' visits and the medicine she must take. When she asks her mother, her mother tells her the medicine and visits are either for allergies or to make sure she grows tall, because her family is usually very short. The medical staff has not had a "slip up" and Kenya has no idea of her diagnosis. She does worry though, because her mother is always worried about germs and her getting sick. Kenya has absorbed her mother's fear and is very afraid of germs, carrying a hand sanitizer with her and turning away when anyone sneezes. Kenya believes that the hand sanitizer can "cure her" just as her grandmother uses salves and herbal medicine for healing.

Kenya's school performance is below average for a child in her age range. She has not yet learned to read and is not doing well with writing skills. Her teacher thought she had noticed some problems with Kenya's pencil grip and mentioned this to her mother at Kenya's fall teacher-parent conference. Kenya's teacher also reported concerns with her sporadic class attendance and fear of germs. Finally, her teacher was concerned that she is experiencing delays in reading and learning to write. Kenya's mother, Lalliana, automatically became defensive, and stated that she believed her daughter fights a lot of colds and that her academic skills will reach the level of other children in her age range by the end of the current academic year. With urging from Kenya's teacher, her mother reluctantly agreed to have a conference with the school psychologist.

The interview with the school psychologist began with a rocky start. Kenya's mother came late and answered many initial questions with monosyllabic, non-committal responses. When asked about her daughter's health and pre-occupation with germs, Kenya's mother paused and then a silence fell. The school psychologist was ready to ask another question, and surprisingly, Kenya's mother began to weep. Lilliana finally broke her silence and told the school psychologist that her daughter had HIV. The school psychologist offered caring and support as she listened to information about Kenya's chronic illness. Lilliana's behavior calmed after sharing information about her worry and fear for her daughter's health. She let the school psychologist know that she expects and reinforces Kenya's use of hand sanitizer and tells her it is a "magic lotion" that will help her grow and ward off evil germs, just like grandma does with her healing potions. Kenya came home right away if her hands cracked. Kenya's grandmother did use a lot of herbs and traditional healing methods, common to her culture in Mexico. The school psychologist listened and respected Kenya's mother's needs to share information and share her ideas for helping her daughter stay healthy. The school psychologist established a very positive relationship with Lilliana.

The school psychologist understood that Lilliana was feeling overwhelmed if there were many people in the room, so the first part of the meeting was with the school nurse, the school psychologist and Lilliana. Information about Kenya's medical condition was shared and they discussed what would happen if Kenya had a nose bleed or an injury involving bleeding at school. In the next part of the meeting, Lillana met with Kenya's teacher and let her know about Kenya's medical condition. Kenya often did not want to play with others at recess or participate in gym, due to her fear of germs. The group agreed on other activities that Kenya could do, since she refused to participate in gym or recess. They talked about her spending time with the reading specialist or with the art teacher during gym and recess. Kenya's teacher again requested an evaluation of Kenya's academic skills, due to her delays in reading and writing. Lilliana reluctantly agreed to the assessment.

The school psychologist met with Kenya and administered a test of intellectual functioning and achievement skills. After scoring the measures, the school psychologist noted a 25 point discrepancy between Kenya's score on the test of intellectual functioning and her performance on the reading comprehension subtest and the writing subtest on the test of her achievement skills. The school psychologist developed a written report highlighting her findings and referred Kenya for services from the school reading specialist and for evaluation by an occupational therapist. Information in the report was shared with Kenya's mother during a meeting, and her mother agreed to both referrals, as long as reading lessons occurred in manner that did not make Kenya "stand out." After this, Kenya's mother signed an Individual Education Plan and met with the school psychologist, the leader of the special education team, the reading specialist, and Kenya's teacher to develop an appropriate plan to facilitate her academic development. Re-evaluation will occur yearly, with re-administration of testing at three year intervals or as necessary.

The school psychologist discussed a possible meeting between herself, the school nurse, Lilliana, and a member of Kenya's medical team. At the meeting, the school psychologist learned that there is a pediatric psychologist or child health psychologist that specializes in working with children with HIV and their families at the nearby children's hospital. Lilliana's mother talked with the pediatric psychologist; however, she did not feel that Kenya should meet with the pediatric psychologist. In time, the pediatric psychologist helped Kenya's mother resolve grief and loss issues related to her daughter's condition and help her process her own guilt, as she too had HIV. In the long run, this referral was very helpful in providing psychological support to Kenya and her mother. The school psychologist also noted that the pediatric psychologist could assist Kenya in reducing her use of hand sanitizer and fears of germs. A further goal is to assist Kenya in becoming more integrated in her community and in developing relationships with her peers.

Case Study 2: Boy with Food Allergies

This case highlights the special needs of a child with multiple types of food allergies, including nuts, eggs, and chocolate in the school setting. This child also had mental health problems, including Attention Deficit Hyperactivity Disorder and Oppositional Defiant Disorder. Finally the child had speech and language deficits. He was in second grade at a private elementary school outside a medium-sized urban area. This young boy saw his pediatrician regularly, and a host of other medical specialists, including a mental health provider in a private practice setting.

One of his first goals in therapy was to reduce his fear of needles and fear of using his epi-pen, should he have a severe allergic reaction. Another goal was to reduce the frequency with which he asked for Benadryl. His fears emanated from a previous negative experience at his doctor's office, where he had to be held down

--- adults held his arms and legs as he laid on a table --- in order to receive a shot from his epi-pen after he mistakenly ate egg products at a peer's birthday party. The boy's therapist elected to use play therapy to help the child express his medical fears and work through his anger and upset over being restrained to receive a shot.

Several play sessions, involving play with medical toys and figures and hospital equipment, were held. During these sessions, the boy had an opportunity to share feelings of anger and helplessness and play through his feelings and upset related to his past traumatic medical experience. In the play room he had control over the outcome of the play. Through play, the therapist also had opportunities to suggest positive ways in which the child could cope with shots should he have to receive a shot in the future. They practiced using the epi-pen on an orange and the little boy was able to learn that the shot was quick and that is was easy to insert the shot into an orange. After the fourth session, the boy told his mother he was less afraid of shots and she would be able to administer a shot to him. Moreover, the frequency with which the boy asked for Benadryl decreased and he was less focused on being exposed to an egg and getting sick at home, school, and at outings with his friends.

At about this time, the mother informed the therapist that the boy was having an evaluation, to rule out Attention-Deficit Hyperactivity Disorder in order to improve his school performance and improve teacher perceptions of him. The boy was apparently having difficulty with outbursts in the classroom, becoming angry when peers talked to or bothered him and at times he refused to talk to his teacher. He said that he refused to talk with her because she did not listen to his report that the children alongside of him were bothering him as he attempted to complete his school assignments.

The evaluation at the local children's hospital indicated that the boy did in fact have Attention Deficit Hyperactivity Disorder as well as Oppositional Defiant Disorder. The boy was seen by a child psychiatrist for a "medication evaluation" and Ritalin was prescribed. In addition, the psychologist received useful recommendations to help the boy improve his behaviors at school. Among these recommendations were: using a daily school-home note to document classroom behavior, seating the boy close to the teacher so that she could monitor his school progress, writing down his homework assignments in a daily planner so he had a record of homework to complete, and utilizing a star chart (reward chart) along with frequent praise for on-task and prosocial behaviors. His mother implemented a reward system at home, where he received 15 more minutes of video game play those days that he was on-task and had a positive day at school.

In order to manage angry and oppositional behaviors, the boy was referred to both the school psychologist and his private practice mental health provider. These providers talked by telephone and reviewed the report developed by the hospital specialty team. They agreed with the diagnoses of Attention-Deficit Hyperactivity Disorder and Oppositional Defiant Disorder. They worked together to implement a school-based reward system, where the boy received prizes at the end of the week if he had eight to ten stars on his star chart. At the school store, run by a local graduate student, children could select prizes for positive behaviors at the end of the week. The boy usually earned a prize at the end of the week.

The school psychologist also suggested that he and his teacher have a special cueing word to alert the boy that he needed to get his behavior on track, when he was being defiant or was significantly off-task. This cue word was "go-time." When the teacher very gently tapped the boy on the shoulder or caught his gaze and said "go-time" he had a reminder to check on his behavior and a chance to "turn his behavior around" before it escalated to a level that was considered negative by the teacher. The special signal worked. Over time he exhibited improved behaviors in the classroom.

In the long-run, there were improvements in the positive nature of teacher-child interactions. The boy was much happier at school and negative behaviors reduced and refusal to talk with the teacher about his behavior completely stopped. The boy became proud of this academic performance and his grades improved from "C's" to "B's." Concomitantly, his relationship with his mother and father improved at home, as they were able to reduce their role as disciplinarians (due to providing discipline for his poor behavior at school).

The boy participated in bi-weekly sessions with his private therapist, where they worked on strategies to help him calm himself. He learned to "count" and "walk away" before becoming angry. Relaxation techniques, such as squeezing out his anger after making a fist, also helped him release his energy and upset feelings in the school setting. He learned to have a checklist to complete his school work and always put his homework in his backpack in his "finished" folder before ending his nightly homework period. He learned to take short breaks, where he did jumping jacks and then returned to his schoolwork, which helped him to complete his school work.

In the classroom and at school, the boy was taught to ask to sit in his favorite chair or in his "calm down" spot so that he could think, relax, and then reduce his angry words. Going to his calm down spot and sitting quietly helped in reducing impulsive, negative responses and reduced conflict with the teacher and the boy and his mother and the boy. Furthermore, over time the boy expressed pride of accomplishment because, "I can calm down and get it together." His self-esteem improved and he appeared happier and satisfied with his ability to "pull my behavior together when I am getting mad."

The intervention involved multiple medical providers and components across the home and school contexts. Evaluation was a key factor in determining diagnoses and planning for behavior change at school. A Section 504 plan was developed to ensure that classroom accommodations were recorded and to ensure that school staff knew the boy needed to eat lunch at a special table in the lunchroom with one other child who had food allergies. The boy became more comfortable around his peers at school, when he reduced his worries and concerns about being exposed to foods he was allergic to at lunch. After a year, the boy was again exposed to eggs, by accident, at a classmate's birthday party, and his mother was able to successfully administer his epi-pen so that he did not experience a severe allergic reaction.

CONCLUSION

An inclusive approach, valuing the opinions of the medical team, parent, teachers, and the child him or herself, may be a way to develop a plan that best "fits" the needs of the child and allows him or her to flourish in school. Accommodations should be considered as actions to promote growth and inclusion, as a way to facilitate the academic, behavioral, social, and emotional development of the child. Additional research is needed to understand the long-term development and "longitudinal consequences" (Halfon *et al.*, 2012, p. 35) of academic and school development and achievement for children with special needs.

Halfon *et al.*, (2012) discussed the initiative or study at the Eunice K. Shriver National Institute for Child Health and Human Development (NICHD) as one project that may provide information about child achievement and development from birth through adulthood. The NICHD is conducting a study with 100,000 children from preconception to age twenty. The results of this longitudinal study will provide a depth perspective of child development and information about ways that child-environment interactions shape child development. Obtaining a comprehensive view of child development is important for learning about ways to meet the educational and developmental needs of children so that all can develop to their fullest potential. Assessment of protective and risk factors impacting development and academic progress for children with medical conditions within the group participating in the aforementioned study will provide a longitudinal perspective on factors that can impact educational and social-emotional functioning for children who have chronic illnesses.

ACKNOWLEDGEMENTS

None declared.

CONFLICT OF INTEREST

The author confirms that this chapter contents have no conflict of interest.

REFERENCES

Adler, J., Raju, S., Beveridge, A. S., Wang, S., Zhu, J., & Zimmerman, E. M. (2008). College adjustment in University of Michigan students with Crohn's and Colitis. *Inflammatory Bowel Disease, 14*(9), 1281-1286.

Armstrong, T. (2012). *Neurodiversity in the classroom: Strength-based strategies to help students with special needs succeed in school and life*. Alexandria, VA: ASCD Publishers.

Barraclough, C., & Machek, G. (2010). School psychologists' role concerning children with chronic illnesses in schools. *Journal of Applied School Psychology, 26*(2), 132-148.

Bitsko, R. H., Visser, S. N., Schieve, L. A., Ross, D. S., Thurman, D. J., & Perou, R. (2009). Unmet health care needs among CSHCN with neurologic conditions. *Pediatrics, 124,* S343-S351.

Boulet, S. L., Boyle, C. A., & Schieve, L. A. (2009). Health care use and health and functional impact of developmental disabilities among U.S. children, 1997-2005. *Adolescent Medicine, 163*(1), 19-26.

Clay, D. L. (2004). *Helping schoolchildren with chronic health conditions: A practical guide.* The Guilford Practical Intervention in School Series. New York: Guilford Press.

Forrest, C. B., Bevans, K. B., Riley, A. W., Crespo, R., & Louis, T. A. (2011). School outcomes of children with special health care needs. *Pediatrics, 128*, 303-312.

Gargiulo, R., & Kilgo, J. L. (2012). *An Introduction to Young Children with Special Needs: Birth Through Age Eight: Fourth Edition.* Cengage Learning.

Guilford, R., & Upton, G. (2006). *Special Educational Needs.* New York: Routledge.

Halfon, N., Houtrow, A., Larson, K., & Newacheck, P. W. (2012). The changing landscape of disability in childhood. *Future of Children, 22*(1), 13-42.

Individuals with Disabilities Education Act of 2004, P.L. 108-446.

Irwin, M. K., & Elam, M. (2011). Are we leaving children with chronic illness behind? *Physical Disabilities: Education and Related Services. 30*(2), 67-80.

Logan, D. E., Simons, L. E., Stein, M. J., & Chastain, L. (2008). School impairment in adolescents with chronic pain. *Journal of Pain, 9*(5), 407-416.

Madaus, J. W., & Shaw, S. F. (2004). Section 504: Differences in the regulations for secondary and post-secondary education. Intervention in the *School and Clinic, 40*(2), 81-87.

Nabors, L., Akin-Little, A., Little, S., & Iobst, E. (2008). Teachers' knowledge about chronic illnesses. For the mini-series: Psychology's contribution to education: Improving educational opportunities for all children. *Psychology in the Schools, 45*, 217-226.

Power, T. J., & Bradley-Klug, K. L. (2013). *Pediatric school psychology: Conceptualization, applications, and strategies for leadership development. In the school-based practice in action series.* New York: Routledge.

Shaw, S. R., & McCabe, P. C. (2008). Hospital-to-school transition for children with chronic illness: Meeting the new challenges of an evolving healthcare system. *Psychology in the Schools, 45*(1), 74-87.

Suris, J. C., Michaud, P. A., & Viner, R. (2004). The adolescent with a chronic condition. Part I: Developmental issues. *Archives of Disease in Childhood, 89*(10), 938-942.

U. S. Department of Education (2007). *Free appropriate public education for students with disabilities: Requirements under Section 504 of the Rehabilitation Act of 1973.* Washington D. C.: Office for Civil Rights.

World Health Organization. International Classification of Functioning, Disability, and Health (2001). Geneva Switzerland: World Health Organization.

Send Orders for Reprints to reprints@benthamscience.net

CHAPTER 6

Facilitating Adherence to the Child's Medical Regimen

Laura A. Nabors[*]

Health Education Program, School of Human Services, University of Cincinnati, 468 Dyer Hall, Mail Location 0068, Cincinnati, Ohio, OH 45221-0068, USA

Abstract: This chapter addresses adherence, which is loosely defined as following the medical regimen, for a child with a chronic illness. Children with chronic illnesses often have complex regimens. They and their parents can benefit from support for taking their medications as well as for following dietary and exercise recommendations. Use of rewards and reminder notes and calendars can be helpful tools for improving recall of the multiple steps of a medical regimen. Adolescence may be a special risk period for poor adherence and careful monitoring of adherence at this stage, and referral when needed, can be supportive for families and the adolescent him- or herself. Education and improving the health knowledge of the child and his or her parents and encouraging a team approach may be other factors that strengthen adherence to complex medication schedules and medical regimens.

Keywords: Adherence, adherence barriers, adolescent adherence, facilitating adherence, medical compliance, medication schedules.

INTRODUCTION

An important area in which to increase expertise is helping the child and family adhere to the pediatrician's recommendations. This means developing a plan or skills for the child and caregiver(s) to follow all directions provided by the health care team, typically chiefly represented by the child's doctor, so that the child experiences success in terms of medical management and illness outcomes. Children with medical conditions often have complex medication regimens, which can make adherence challenging. Reasons for a lack of adherence include side effects of medications, depression, inability to understand medical instructions, and a lack of support from family members. In contrast, factors that

---

*Address correspondence to **Laura A. Nabors:** Health Education Program, School of Human Services, University of Cincinnati, 468 Dyer Hall, Mail Location 0068, Cincinnati, Ohio, OH 45221-0068, USA; Tel: 513-556-5537; Fax: 513-556-3898; E-mail: naborsla@ucmail.uc.edu

facilitate adherence are having a positive attitude about the treatment or regimen being successful and support from family (DiMatteo *et al.,* 2000). Monitoring charts, pill organizers, pill counts, and reward systems may assist the child in keeping up with his or her medication regimen. Children who have medical conditions often need to change their eating or exercise patterns, which is another area for "adherence" or area to work on, in terms of complying with the medical regimen.

Children who have chronic illnesses adhere to their medical regimens approximately 50% of the time (DiMatteo *et al.,* 2000; Rapoff, 1999). Adherence may differ across various aspects of the medical regimen. For example, children with cystic fibrosis may be less likely to adhere to or follow dietary instructions and recommendations, whereas they may be more likely to adhere to chest physical therapy recommendations, which help to clear their airways. Modi and Quittner (2006) mentioned that several factors may influence adherence, including recall of the instructions (*i.e.*, forgetting), the difficulty of the regimen, oppositional behaviors on the part of the patient/child, child and parent knowledge about the illness and what to do, having enough time to complete a complex regimen, side effects of medications, lack of support from family members and communication between the doctor or health care team and the patient (child) and his or her caregivers. At the child level, a host of different factors, such as dislike of medications or difficulty with pill swallowing, may also impact medication adherence. Use of daily diaries may be one way to learn about the complex factors that affect child and parent adherence to different parts of the medical regimen, under different circumstances (Modi & Quittner, 2006).

Another difficult condition, in terms of adherence, is obstructive sleep apnea. The initial treatment for this is a tonsillectomy and/or adenoidectomy (Marcus *et al.,* 2006). If these treatments are unsuccessful or if the child is obese and has poor respiratory tone, then the symptoms of obstructive sleep apnea will persist. A next level treatment is continuous or bi-level positive airway pressure (PAP) therapy. These children wear masks and headgear and receive extra oxygen to help with breathing during the night. Many children with obstructive sleep apnea drop out of treatment with the masks, because they are not easy to wear. In their study, Marcus *et al.,* (2006) found that use of PAP therapy was successful for a group of about twenty children with obstructive sleep apnea. Mean use of the PAP machines was about 5 hours (Standard Deviation about 2.5 hours). Non-adherence was defined as use of the PAP machine for less than three hours per night.

Those who did "stick with" or continue using the PAP machine had positive outcomes according to parent report. For instance, children were sleeping better, not falling asleep as frequently in school if they were using the PAP system. Parents also stated that children spent less time snoring and were increasingly well-rested after a period of being treated with the PAP machine. Marcus *et al.*, (2006) recommended that in order to gauge adherence most accurately, researchers should use multiple measures, such as hours of use of the PAP machine and parent and child report of adherence, in order to accurately assess adherence to wearing the PAP system.

ADOLESCENCE: A RISK PERIOD FOR POOR ADHERENCE

Adolescents may be a risk group for poor adherence (Gardiner & Dvorkin, 2006; Rapoff, 1999). In order to reach adolescents, and influence positive attitudes toward adherence, the health care provider may want to speak about things that are important to adolescents, such as social factors, appearance, and involvement in activities (Yeo & Sawyer, 2005). Additionally, it is advisable for the medical team to listen to barriers proposed by adolescents and concomitantly involve the adolescent in decision-making and discussion of adherence planning. Ensuring that the adolescent can successfully develop a routine to manage his or her illness or implement adherence steps in his or her everyday life are other important factors to consider when designing plans to maximize adherence.

Dziuban *et al.*, (2010) assessed adherence in sixty adolescents and young adults (between 12 – 20 years) with cystic fibrosis. They reported that this was an important group to study, because as medications increased and as the disease progressed there was a decline in adherence to the medical regimen. A questionnaire was designed for this study to examine barriers to adherence. They also examined attitudes related to adherence. Their findings indicated that older patients in their sample were in relatively poorer health than younger ones. Often, aging was related to negative progression of the disease, which, in turn, was related to low levels of adherence. Barriers to adherence included time management, there being "too much" to do to allow for effective monitoring, and forgetting. Younger adolescents could also feel embarrassed about having cystic fibrosis. Moreover, youth who felt that their freedom was restricted due to their illness were less likely to adhere, as were those who were struggling with a complex (very complicated) medical regimen. The adolescent and young adult years also may be stressful if children are "tired of their disease" and begin to have treatment fatigue and take breaks from following their treatment regimen due to this fatigue. It is important for physicians and the medical team to stress the importance of adherence with their patients, when symptoms are flaring or worsening, in order to bolster their resolve to cope with and follow their medical regimen. Questions to ask adolescents include their perceptions of loss of freedom related to their illness and the management routine, their beliefs about their ability to follow their regimen, and their notions about whether their medical team is supportive of their efforts.

MEDICATION ADHERENCE

Gardiner and Dvorkin (2006) discussed ideas for assisting children and their caregivers as well as pediatricians with improving medication compliance. For children and caregivers, some of their recommendations were to: (1) take the medication at the same time each day, (2) incorporate medical care into family routines, (3) use a calendar to track dosing and other key adherence behaviors, (4) use of reminders [*e.g.*, notes, alarms on cell phones, watches], (5) build positive family support, and (6) use rewards for adhering to doctor's recommendations. Gardiner and Dvorkin suggested ideas for pediatricians too, which included: (1) discussing adherence with the child and family, (2) using educational materials, (3) reviewing tips for adherence during medical appointments, (4) prescribing medications requiring 1 to 2 doses daily [more can be too complex for families], (5) discussing issues related to medication safety, and (6) reminding other health professionals to stress the importance of regular medication regimens and adherence to all aspects of the child's medical regimen. Adherence is assessed in a number of ways including use of blood assays, pill counts, appointment records (*e.g.*, keeping appointments), and self-report by patients (*i.e.*, children and parents) as well as report by doctors.

Dean *et al.,* (2010) reviewed 17 studies, all of which were controlled trials, examining the impact of interventions to improve medication adherence. Their findings indicated that behavioral interventions, such as monitoring, pill counts, rewards for taking medicines, *etc.* were effective interventions for improving medication adherence by children who had chronic illnesses. In contrast, educational interventions were not deemed effective. A behavioral intervention combined with the educational components might improve the impact of educational interventions. Overall, however, Dean *et al.,* (2010) concluded that questions remain, because research needs to be conducted with children at different stages of development and research needs to be conducted with children who have very poor adherence to medication regimens.

Children with epilepsy may be at risk for poor adherence to their medication management. This poor adherence can contribute to seizure onset. Modi *et al.,* (2008) discussed the use of medication event monitoring systems or MEMS caps to track pill taking in children with epilepsy. The MEMS caps keep a record, which can be downloaded to a computer, of the number of times the medication bottle is opened. Modi *et al.,* (2008) used MEMS caps to track medication management of children newly diagnosed with epilepsy during their first month since diagnosis. Only 23% of the children and their parents/caregivers displayed complete adherence to the medication regimen. In general, about 76-80% of the children and parents in their sample adhered to the new medical regimen in the first month after the child's diagnosis. Interestingly, if parents were married then child adherence improved, relative to parents who were single. There were not gender differences in adherence. These researchers also examined what they termed, "white coat compliance." This occurs when there is, "… improved adherence that occurs a short time before a clinic visit (p. e961, Modi *et al.,* 2008). They examined adherence rates one and five days prior to the appointment and found that adherence during these times was not different from adherence during the rest of the first month after diagnosis.

Janicke *et al.,* (2009) conducted a pilot study to assess the impact of victimization and support on treatment adherence, chiefly medication management adherence, for 38 children with Irritable Bowel Syndrome, between the ages of 7 to 19 years. Most of the youth in their sample had ulcerative colitis or Crohn's disease. It is noteworthy that similar to many studies, the developmental age range of youth in this study was broad and this broad age range could have impacted study findings. The reason for this is that differences could be a result of developmental influences (*e.g.*, change in child attitudes at different ages) rather than positive or negative aspects of disease management or complexity of medical regimen. In their sample, they reported that adherence to treatment was good or high. They examined parent, child, and physician reports of medication adherence. They found that these three sources provided related or similar ratings. Their findings indicated that when social support was perceived to be low, then medication adherence was adversely impacted by peer victimization experience. Children's perceptions of support from others were related to positive management. Perceptions of support from significant others moderated the negative influence of being a peer victim on adherence.

A group that may have a great deal of difficulty with adherence to a medication regimen is children with HIV. Dolezal *et al.,* (2003) examined self-report of 48 pairs of parents and children for child adherence to medical regimens for HIV. Children with HIV have to take multiple medications with side effects (both short- and long-term), are often fearful of stigma related to discovery of their condition, and face regular barriers to adherence, such as forgetting and not having enough time to follow a complicated regimen. These authors mentioned that another barrier to learning about and planning for non-adherence is that parents and children may not report problems with following the medical regimen because they "want to look positive" for their doctors and medical team. If this type of bias occurs, then children and caregivers do not get the support that they need. Medication adherence in HIV management is difficult to assess and parent and child reports may not concur, especially during the adolescent period. In their study over one-third of the dyads showed a lack of agreement about child adherence to medication regimes and medical management. Dolezal and colleagues suggested that a lack of agreement between child and parent/caregiver report of adherence might indicate a need to intervene, in order to improve adherence efforts.

POOR COMMUNICATION AS A BARRIER TO ADHERENCE

Another reason that children may not adhere is that they do not understand what to do, related to poor communication or a lack of understanding of the directions or instructions provided by their doctors. Communicative health literacy refers to children's communication with their doctor. It affects patients' abilities to follow through with recommendations and their health outcomes (Berkman *et al*., 2004; Nutbeam, 2000). If a child and his or her caregiver do not communicate well with their doctors or medical team, they both may lack an understanding of what to do, in terms of instructions to follow in order to fulfill the requirements of the child's medical regimen.

Carmona (2006) reported that the health care mission of doctors will be "marginalized" (p. 803) unless communication improves between doctors and their patients. There may be a direct link between improved sharing of information between patients and doctors and positive health outcomes. Nutbeam (2000) and Baker (2006) viewed communicative or oral health literacy, as involving information sharing between the doctor, parent and child; they believed that communication and health outcomes were interrelated. Hence, if a doctor is able to communicate with the child (*i.e.*, there is a high level of doctor-child communication), the child and parent will gain knowledge and share information leading to better diagnosis, recommendations, and health outcomes (Baker, 2006).

One key to improving adherence may be for doctors and health care professionals to have longer conversations with children and caregivers. During these conversations they should encourage questions and allow children and caregivers to review their understanding of the instructions. Parent and child adherence to treatment recommendations may improve when doctor-child communication improves during the visit (Lewis *et al*., 1991; Tates *et al*., 2002). Wissow and Bar-Din Kimel (2002) reported that spending time with the doctor and more attention from the doctor during children's emergency visits for asthma resulted in a very positive health outcome for children – decreased morbidity.

FAMILY FUNCTIONING

Reaching children in their early years, and facilitating good medical management with both children and their caregivers can lead to the development of positive adherence habits and a lifelong pattern of adherence that is associated with positive health outcomes (Davis *et al*., 2001). Family climate and parenting behaviors may be related to adherence for young children. Davis *et al.*, (2001) reported that for young children with Type I Diabetes -- family conflict may be related to lower levels of adherence. On the other hand, "…family cohesion and organization have been associated with better adherence and glycemic control (p. 124, Davis *et al.*, 2001). Participants for the aforementioned research were 55 preschool and elementary school-aged children. These researchers assessed parental warmth, which was associated with improved adherence to the children's diabetes regimen. Conversely, restrictive parenting styles were related to poorer glycemic control. Further study is needed to determine the family variables and parent-child relationship factors determining adherence to the child's medical regimen; this could lead to the development of parent training interventions that would assist caregivers. Moreover, more research is needed with young children, in order to facilitate the development of healthy adherence patterns that may last for a lifetime.

COPING, ADJUSTMENT, AND ADHERENCE

The relations among child and family coping skills and strategies, child and family adjustment to the chronic condition and medical regimen, and subsequent adherence are complex. The relationships among these three factors are multifaceted, dynamic, and changing – based upon contextual factors. Research has made a significant, undeniable contribution to guiding clinical practice and has pointed to the need for documentation of interventions, so that there is an evidence base to guide clinical practice. Fig. (**1**) presents one representation of the relations among factors that impact coping, child and family adjustment to a child's illness and its management, and adherence to the child's medical regimen.

This complex relationship is hard to depict in a two dimensional figure (see Fig. **1**). In general, coping skills and child and family characteristics and experiences are related to adjustment to the child's illness and all its implications, including attitudes that the family can and will cope with the demands of the child's medical regimen. In turn, these variables are related to adherence. However, adherence is impacted by many factors and even if the family follows the regimen perfectly, measures such as blood assays, may provide a skewed picture, indicating that disease management is not optimal or is even poor. This is discouraging and can contribute to worry and concern, leading to feelings of hopelessness with following the regimen, because "best efforts" do not result in success. This can lead to a lack of coping attempts or child or parent anxiety and depression. This may mean that adherence efforts and illness management take a downturn.

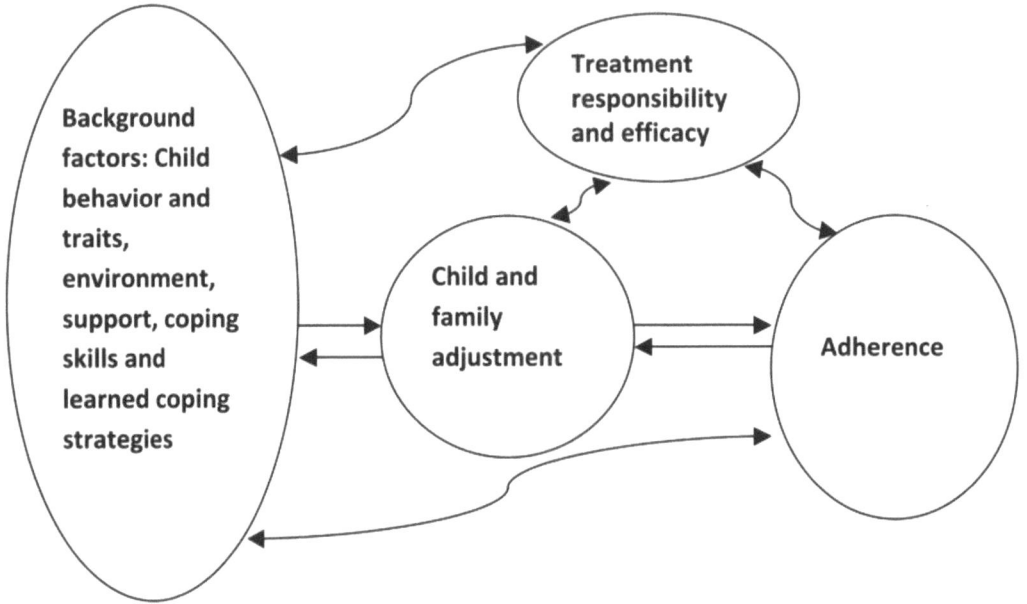

Figure 1: Outline of a model of factors related to adherence.

For any number of reasons, the pattern can reverse and adherence and coping can improve. The relationships are not linear, but are multi-faceted and impacted by any number of attitudinal variables (for both child and caregiver), contextual variables (*e.g.*, support at school from the teacher), and disease course and factors impacting disease progression. The factors in Fig. (**1**) have reciprocal, evolving influences on each other, making the relationship between coping and adherence difficult to assess and interpret, as evidenced by the curved lines in Fig. (**1**). Additionally, the complex relations among the multiple factors influencing adherence challenge the clinician to understand the literature in his or her field and to gain a thorough understanding of the child, family, medical team, the child's illness, and the prescribed medical regimen, in order to provide recommendations that will facilitate high efficacy for feelings of treatment responsibility, leading to adherence and, ultimately, positive health outcomes.

Compas *et al.,* (2012) wrote extensively about child coping in their article in the *Annual Review of Clinical Psychology*. Information in this manuscript indicated that coping efforts and adherence are intertwined, and that disengagement from coping, such as what can occur if feelings of learned helplessness to impact disease management persist, can negatively affect adherence and health outcomes over time. If the child or family relinquishes control and does not implement coping strategies and stops following the medical regimen, long-term prognosis for adherence and disease management is relatively poor. The good news, however, is that many factors can influence an upturn in positive attitude such as, feeling one can cope, increased feelings of treatment responsibility and efficacy for management of the disease, and improved adherence behaviors. This offers many avenues for clinicians to intervene (*e.g.*, making environmental changes, working with the child to help him or her feel less anxious, and implementing psychoeducational strategies to teach and empower caregivers and children). A model of coping, adjustment and adherence can be positive and empowering by nature, as there are many points for intervention. There are innumerable positive strategies to improve child and family feelings of resilience and hope so that they can adjust to the child's illness and adhere to the child's medical regimen. As a discipline, mental health has only scratched the surface of these many positive coping strategies and much more research and study is needed to determine ways to improve positive thinking and feelings of efficacy for coping will illness.

As mentioned, communication with the medical team is critical (Caromona, 2006). Communication is impacted by child and family feelings of empowerment to effectively cope with the disease as well as physician and medical team efforts to reach and communicate with the child. If these communication channels break down or are in dis-repair, then the mental health clinician can play a key role as a mediator, in re-opening communication channels. This can improve child and parent skills for making positive appraisals of their situation and their abilities to tackle the complexities of following the child's medical regimen.

Borrowing strategies from positive psychology and improving feelings of optimism and self-efficacy for the child and family also may positively impact adherence behaviors at the child and family level (Bandura, 1994; Seligman, 2002; Seligman & Csikszentmihalyi, 2000). Application of Gardiner and

Dvorkin's (2006) ideas for improving adherence can also start a backward chain, causing a positive evolution in attitude about the illness and coping, thereby alleviating feelings of child and caregiver anxiety and depression related to the stress of coping with a chronic illness (see Fig. **1**). Next, a review of some case studies is presented to emphasize key coping processes and interventions that might boost adherence efforts for the child and his or her family.

CASE STUDY: RENAL TRANSPLANTATION

John was an eight-year-old boy experiencing renal failure. He had participated in Make-A-Wish and had a wonderful visit to Disneyworld with his parents and sister. He was on the kidney transplant list, but hopes for a kidney were slim. At the last minute, a kidney became available. John received a transplant. He had prepared himself for the disappointment of not having a transplant and having to remain on dialysis for the rest of his life. He was unprepared for the major surgery and the complex treatment regimen that followed the surgery. His parents were in the same situation. They did not have knowledge of the complex regimen that would follow and the struggle John would endure as his body adjusted to a new organ.

The surgery was complex and John remained in the pediatric intensive care unit (PICU) for weeks after transplantation. His family lived two hours away. He had a sibling and his parents were working, making visiting every day impossible. As his parents' visits declined John became less adherent to his medication regime. An attending physician in the PICU contacted a child psychologist working in the hospital to work with John to relieve stress and feelings of homesickness that often accompany young children who must remain in the PICU for an extended period of time. The physician, Dr. Cramer, described John's condition as, "PICU-itis. This reaction is accompanied by sadness, and sometimes anger and noncompliance – such as refusing to eat or take medications or fluids." Dr. Cramer asked the pediatric psychologist to help relieve feelings of boredom, sadness and help John adhere or go along with taking his medications post-transplant.

The psychologist came up with a multifaceted plan to assist John with his PICU-itis. First, child life was contacted. A video game station was installed in John's room and was going to remain there until he transferred to a step-down unit. A child life specialist would visit John. Plans were made to have a high school student, volunteering with the child life team, to come and play board and video games with John three days a week.

The pain team was contacted for consultation. They decided John would receive an intravenous line to administer his medications – in a titrated dosage– through a push button when he needed them. The medications were set so that he could only receive the correct dosage. It was evident that John relished the feeling of control over his pain medications – he was bedridden and this was the one thing, besides ordering what he wanted to eat, that was within his control. Every day the pain specialist "checked in" with John to see how he was doing with his pain. This intervention did John a world of good, as he began to feel responsible for his "getting well."

Pictures of his parents were placed in his bed stand and on the railings on either side of his bed. The psychologist met with his parents, during their bi-weekly visit day, and recorded their voices on an iPad, and John had their voices and messages stored in this device and could replay their well wishes. Daily phone calls to his mother, prior to lunch and dinner, helped encourage him to eat and were related to improved compliance with medical rounds where residents were checking his stitches and stomach to see how he was healing. Before these "pep talks" and calls John was becoming obstreperous when the medical team came for rounds. After the calls and pep talks, John started to tolerate rounds better.

The physicians also adopted an "ask John what to look at next plan" during rounds. Residents and physicians always asked John what he would like "looked at next." In this way, John had control over what they checked when they came by. Sometimes this meant that the resident or physician had to return several times to examine John, but the exam always happened, and without a struggle. With John's help, it was easier to check his progress and the physicians and residents had a better view of his surgical site. They also began showing him what they would do using a toy dog before changing his bandages or making any change to his routine care. The dog was called Little Johnny and all procedures where demonstrated on the dog before being completed with John. This process enhanced John's knowledge of what was going to happen and reduced his anxiety.

The child psychologist visited John 2 times per week. During these visits, John and the psychologist played games and he had an opportunity to share his feelings. Over time, John was able to express feelings of fear and loss of control related to his medical condition and all the procedures he had endured. He talked about being at his "Make-a-Wish at Disney, and then I had to come home from my wish and have a bad time." The psychologist was able to allow John to express his feelings. He was able to do this in a safe environment, processing feelings related to medical trauma in his own time and in his own way.

After some time had passed, John graduated from game play to drawing, and he and the therapist made a coping book describing what had happened to John and how he was coping with his new kidney. John defined coping as, "Getting along with it (the kidney) and accepting a new part of me." He talked about how hard it was to accept a new part of him (new body part) that brought him pain and made it necessary for him to, "take all this yucky medicine." His drawings, at first uncontrolled, became detailed and told the story of a boy learning to accept his new body part and doing well with it. As the book progressed in a positive manner so did John's acceptance of his transplant and his compliance with his medical regimen.

In addition to expressing his feelings, John received stickers on a success chart for complying with his medication regimen. For every three check marks, signaling a successful day of adherence to his medication regimen, John received extra game time with someone from child life. He also was able to win toys and books to keep in his room and play with. The nurses' relationships with John improved as he experienced "winning" rewards for good behavior and began to feel responsible for and believe in his ability to help himself get well by adhering to his medical regimen.

After three weeks in the PICU, John was moved to the regular unit. He began to heal and accept the transplant, where at first it was a "touch and go" situation due to his lack of adherence. He came to accept the medications and daily routine of taking care of his new kidney. He was able to make new friends to support him –

in terms of hospital staff. He looked forward to his parents' visits and seeing his sister. After two weeks, John received cards from his classmates. This seemed a boost to his self-esteem, so the pediatric psychologist arranged a conference call where John could talk with his classmates at school.

Soon after John moved to the hospital floor, a teacher began coming from school to help John make up his homework. John looked forward to her visits and keeping up with his school work. He did well with reading and asked for extra books to read. Soon, John asked to write his own story of a boy who missed school and got well with his new kidney. John sang happily to himself as he illustrated his story, with his favorite "power" colors to show him getting well and strong as every day he, "got better and got more used to the nice kidney inside me." Thus, over time, the valence of his situation changed. He began to believe a good thing happened, "getting a new kidney so I wouldn't have to go to dialysis anymore."

After another three weeks John returned home. He continued to see the pediatric psychologist at regular clinic visits as his post-transplant recovery was followed by the renal team. John was able to return to the school environment and routine successfully. His grades remained good and at one year his body was successfully adapting to the "new kidney" post-transplant. John even began taking responsibility for documenting his successes on his chart and reminding his parents when it was time to take "his kidney medicines." John's depression and anxiety decreased.

As can be seen from the case example, John thrived on being involved in his care and being a decision-maker. The care plan in place while he was in the hospital allowed him to practice making decisions and provide input, without bearing the full weight of decision making and while receiving support and rewards for the key role he played in enhancing his own recovery and wellness (Wills *et al.*, 1996). It is important to involve the child, and often his or her family members, in adherence planning and decisions about child medical care. Some children may need to experience a sense of control in order to improve their sense of responsibility for their treatment, which may bolster self-efficacy for coping with the rigors of their medical regimen.

The *Decision-Making Involvement (DMI) Scale* (Miller & Harris, 2012) measures child feelings of control and family communication. This measure may help practitioners to gauge a child's need for involvement in decision-making about his or her medical care. This measure is completed by parents and can inform providers about the child's need for increasing involvement in decision-making and responsibility for his or her medical care. This measure was developed for children with diabetes, asthma, and cystic fibrosis, but questions for this measure can be adapted for children with other types of chronic illnesses. Scores on the *DMI* Scale are associated with locus of control. When children feel in control of their recovery and wellness their self-efficacy for adhering to their medical regimen can improve, thereby leading to better health outcomes. This scale bears further testing to determine its utility for children in different ethnic groups who have different types of illnesses (Miller & Harris, 2012).

Table **1** presents some ideas for helping a child adhere to complex medical regimens to build his or her self-confidence and internal locus of control for being able to cope with his or her illness and concomitant medical regimen.

Table 1:   Ideas for Facilitating Child Adherence

Idea	Intervention(s)
Increase child decision-making.	Use an interview or questionnaire to determine child decision-making and determine steps for improving their input into their medical care.
Improve feelings of efficacy for disease management.	Praise the child for being involved and asking questions; use reward charts to build confidence for adherence behaviors; allow the child to self-administer pain and other medications when possible.
Increase communication with the family and medical team.	Have the medical team ask the child questions and allow the child to present ideas about his or her regimen and care. Family meetings between the medical team, child and family can improve communication and enhance child involvement.
Employ multiple measurement tools to understand adherence phenomena.	Use self-report, pill counts, assays and observations to gain a picture of factors impacting adherence.

Enhancing child involvement in decision–making and thus improving locus of control and self-efficacy for self-management of health routines can improve child feelings of self-confidence and improve adherence. This may result in increased hope, which in the long term also can foster resilience in children.

Improving feelings of strength can assist children in bouncing back from illness and gaining momentum for a developmental trajectory marked by positive functioning. When referring to resilience, a definition is having the abilities or resources to overcome life challenges and stresses that might normally impede a child's progress along a "normal" or positive developmental trajectory (Masten, 2001; Masten *et al.*, 1999). As such, increasing knowledge about adherence and coping has the potential to contribute to literature being amassed related to fostering resilience in children and their families.

Resilient children may be better able to face adversity in the future and thus continue to have strong resources for coping with the progressive nature of many chronic illnesses. Increasing knowledge about resilient functioning in youth and their families can assist child mental health providers in developing interventions and programs to facilitate adaptation. Research is needed on the interplay among the various aspects of adherence behaviors and resilient attitudes, to shed light on the dynamic interactions between these factors. More information is needed on the developmental course of resilience as the child or adolescent grows and copes with chronic medical conditions (Le Brocque *et al.,* 2010), as well as clinical efforts to promote health-related adherence and enhanced feelings of an internal locus of control over one's health. This research will illuminate the pathways through which youth and their families can overcome risk, demonstrate resilience, and achieve optimal health and well-being.

CONCLUSION

In this chapter, key aspects of adherence were reviewed. Suggestions for children and families and physicians were provided. In our case example, it was evident that feelings of self-efficacy and responsibility over "becoming well" inspired a young transplant patient to become more resilient in terms of coping with his kidney transplant. This example illustrated the evolving, interacting relationships between child and family characteristics, adjustment to illness and medical care regimens, and improved adherence. Ultimately, adherence to the medical regimen can result in improved health outcomes. This may circle back, and in the long run improve coping with a severe illness as it progresses and when the child must cope with the waxing and waning symptoms accompanying the course of the illness.

Tips for enhancing adherence and boosting child involvement in his or her medical regimen include having the child "help" with decision-making and rewarding the child and encouraging his or her involvement in his or her self-care. In addition, incorporating the medical regimen into daily routines and making it "a part of life" can improve acceptance of and adherence to medical regimens. In the future, research is needed to inform clinical interventions that will advance positive outcomes for young children and adolescents who have chronic illnesses. Moreover, further knowledge is needed about the relations among various contextual factors (such as coping in the classroom and other settings) and child and family characteristics in order to gain further knowledge about ways to improve adherence to the medical regimen across the myriad of settings in which a child and family functions.

ACKNOWLEDGEMENTS

None declared.

CONFLICT OF INTEREST

The author confirms that this chapter contents have no conflict of interest.

REFERENCES

Baker, D. W. (2006). The meaning and measure of health literacy. *Journal of General Internal Medicine, 21*, 878-883.

Bandura, A. (1994). Self-efficacy. In V. S. Ramachaudran (Ed.), *Encyclopedia of human behavior* (Vol. 4, pp. 71-81). New York: Academic Press. (Reprinted in H. Friedman [Ed.], *Encyclopedia of mental health*. San Diego: Academic Press, 1998).

Berkman, N. D., DeWalt, D. A., Pignone, M. P., Sheridan, S. L., Lohr, K. N., Lux, L., *et al.* (January, 2004). *Literacy and health outcomes. Summary, Evidence Report/Technology Assessment No. 87* (Prepared by RTI International – University of North Carolina Evidence-based Practice Center under Contract No. 290-02-0016). AHRQ Publication No. 04-E007-1. Rockville, MD: Agency for Healthcare Research and Quality.

Carmona, R. H. (2006). Health literacy: A national priority. *Journal of General Internal Medicine, 21*, 803.

Compas, B. E., Jaser, S. S., Dunn, M. J., Rodriquez, E. M. (2012). Coping with chronic illness in childhood and adolescence. *Annual Review of Clinical Psychology, 8*, 455-480.

Davis, C. L., Delamater, A. M., Shaw, K. H., LaGreca, A. M., Eidson, M. S., Perez-Rodriguez, J. E., & Nemery, R. (2001). Brief report: Parenting styles, regimen adherence, and glycemic control in 4- to 10-year-old children with diabetes. *Journal of Pediatric Psychology, 26*(2), 123-129.

Dean, A. J., Walters, J., & Hall, A. (2010). A systematic review of interventions to enhance medication adherence in children and adolescents with chronic illness. *Archives of Disease in Childhood, 95*, 717-723.

DiMatteo, M. R., Lepper, H. S., & Croghan, T. W. (2000). Depression is a risk factor for noncompliance with medical treatment: Meta-analysis of the effects of anxiety and depression on patient adherence. *Archives of Internal Medicine, 160*, 2102-2107.

Dolezal, C., Mellins, C., Brackis-Cott, E., & Abrams, E. J. (2003). The reliability of reports of medical adherence from children with HIV and their adult caregivers. *Journal of Pediatric Psychology, 28*(5), 355-361.

Dziuban, E. J., Saab-Abazeed, L., Chaudhry, S. R., Streetman, D. S., & Nasr, S. Z. (2010). Identifying barriers to treatment adherence and related attitudinal patterns in adolescents with cystic fibrosis. *Pediatric Pulmonology, 45*, 450-458.

Gardiner, P., & Dvorkin, L. (2006). Promoting medication adherence in children. *American Family Physician, 74*(5), 793-798.

Janicke, D. M., Gray, W. N., Kahhan, N. A., Follansbee-Junger, K. W., Marciel, K. K., Storch, E. A., & Jolley, C. D. (2009). Brief report: The association between peer victimization, prosocial support, and treatment adherence in children and adolescents with inflammatory bowel disease. *Journal of Pediatric Psychology, 34*(7), 769-773.

Le Brocque, R. M., Hendrikz, J., & Kenardy, J. A. (2010). The course of post-traumatic stress in children: Examination of recovery trajectories following traumatic injury. *Journal of Pediatric Psychology, 35*, 637-645.

Lewis, C. C., Pantell, R. H., & Sharp, L. (1991). Increasing patient knowledge, satisfaction, and involvement: Randomized trial of a communication intervention. *Pediatrics, 88*, 351-358.

Marcus, C. L., Rosen, G., Davidson-Ward, S. L., Halbower, A. C., Sterni, L., Lutz, J., Stading, P. J., Bolduc, D., & Jordan, J. (2006). Adherence to and effectiveness of positive airway pressure therapy in children with obstructive sleep apnea. *Pediatrics, 117*, e442-e451. doi:10.1542/peds.2005-1634.

Masten, A. S. (2001). Ordinary magic: Resilience processes in development. *American Psychologist, 56*, 227-238.

Masten, A. S., Hubbard, J. J., Gest, S. D., Tellegen, A., Garmezy, N., & Ramirez, M. (1999). Competence in the context of adversity: Pathways to resilience and maladaptation from childhood to late adolescence. *Development and Psychopathology, 11*, 143-169.

McPherson, A. C., Glazebrook, C., Forster, D., James, C., & Smith, A. (2006). A randomized, controlled trial of an interactive educational computer package for children with asthma. *Pediatrics, 117*, 1046-1054.

Miller, V. A., & Harris, D. (2012). Measuring children's decision-making involvement regarding chronic illness management. *Journal of Pediatric Psychology, 37*(3), 292-306.

Modi, A. C., Morita, D. A., & Glauser, T. A. (2008). One-month adherence in children with new-onset epilepsy: White coat compliance does not occur. *Pediatrics, 121*(4), e961-e966. DOI: 10.1542/peds.2007-1960.

Modi, A. C., & Quittner, A. L. (2006). Barriers to treatment adherence for children with cystic fibrosis and asthma: What gets in the way? *Journal of Pediatric Psychology, 31*(8), 846-858.

Nutbeam, D. (2000). Health literacy as a public health goal: A challenge for contemporary health education and communication strategies into the 21st century. *Health Promotion International, 15*, 259-267.

Rapoff, M. A. (1999). *Adherence to pediatric medical regimens.* New York, N.Y.: Kluwer Academic/Plenum Publishers.

Seligman, M. E. P. (2002). Positive psychology, positive prevention, and positive therapy. In C. R. Snyder & S. J. Lopez (Eds). *Handbook of Positive Psychology* (pp. 3-12). New York: Oxford University Press.

Seligman, M. E. P., & Csikszentmihalyi, M. (2000). Positive psychology: An introduction. *American Psychologist, 55*(1), 5-14.

Tates, K. Meeuwesen, L., Elbers, E., & Bensing, J. (2002). I've come for his throat: Roles and identities in doctor-patient-child communication. *Child: Care, Health, and Development, 28*, 109-116.

Wills, T., Blechman, E., & McNamara, G. (1996). Family support, coping and competence. In E. M. Hetherington & E. Blechman (Eds.), *Stress, coping, and resiliency in children and families* (pp. 107-133). Mahwah, N.J.: Lawrence Erlbaum Associates.

Wissow, L. S., & Bar-Din Kimel, M. (2002). Assessing provider-patient-parent communication in the pediatric emergency department. *Ambulatory Pediatrics, 2,* 323-329.

Yeo, M., & Sawyer, S. (2005). ABC of adolescence: Chronic illness and disability. *British Medical Journal, 330*(7493), 721-723.

CHAPTER 7

Parent Adjustment When a Child Experiences a Chronic Illness

Laura A. Nabors[*]

Health Education Program, School of Human Services, University of Cincinnati, 468 Dyer Hall, Mail Location 0068, Cincinnati, Ohio, OH 45221-0068, USA

Abstract: This chapter reviews literature associated with parent adjustment when a child has a chronic illness. This is an important topic, because an ill child is a terrible stressor for the vast majority of parents. There are, of course, the emotional strains, as well as the burden of providing care and the financial burden that can come with the child's chronic illness. Parental reactions can trigger child reactions, such that supporting the parent is a means of supporting the child as well as the family unit. Parent anxiety, depression, and somatic complaints can impact child adjustment and emotional functioning. Being a single parent can also be a risk factor. Social and financial support may be resilience factors for parents, whereas poor family functioning prior to the onset of the child's illness is a potential risk factor for smooth family functioning. A multifaceted plan for supporting parents, the family and child, may be a protective factor for ensuring positive outcomes if a family had been coping poorly before the onset of the child's illness. Continuing to monitor parent functioning is an important goal for ensuring that parents have the support they need to deal with the significant stress of a child's illness.

Keywords: Caregiving burden, emotional stress, parental adjustment, parent depression, single parents, supporting parents.

INTRODUCTION

Parent functioning when a child has a chronic illness can be marked by resilience. At the same time, some parents may be at risk for stress and problems with psychosocial or emotional functioning (Cousino & Hazen, 2013; Dewey & Crawford, 2007). After reviewing the literature, Coffee (2006) suggested that some parents may experience stress and strain as they worry about the welfare of their child and their family unit. They also may worry about expenses, as even

*Address correspondence to Laura A. Nabors: Health Education Program, School of Human Services, University of Cincinnati, 468 Dyer Hall, Mail Location 0068, Cincinnati, Ohio, OH 45221-0068, USA; Tel: 513-556-5537; Fax: 513-556-3898; E-mail: naborsla@ucmail.uc.edu

with insurance, it is costly to care for a child who has a chronic illness. Brown *et al.,* (2008) suggested that parent functioning may inadvertently influence child stress and ability to cope well with his or her illness. Consideration of the mutual or reciprocal influence of child adjustment on the parent and *vice versa* should be considered when conceptualizing the relationship between parent and child adjustment when a child has a chronic illness (Brown *et al.*, 2008; Friedman *et al.*, 2004).

Chernoff *et al.,* (2002) assessed the effectiveness of a supportive intervention to improve child adjustment and decrease mental health problems in children. Child life specialists worked with children to help them accept themselves and improve their self-esteem. Mothers were referred for mentoring from a network of mothers of a child who had the same condition. Children were diagnosed with Type 1 Diabetes, sickle cell anemia, cystic fibrosis, and moderate to severe asthma. One hundred and thirty-six mother-child dyads were examined and mothers and children provided self-report data about child functioning and mental health. Children ranged in age from 7 to 11 years. As a fidelity check, pediatricians and social workers met with child life specialists and mothers to ensure that the intervention was being implemented as planned. Participants were assigned to the intervention group or a comparison group that received treatment as usual, which included being connected to mothers of children with the same types of illnesses. Dose of the intervention was assessed, and was measured as the number of minutes, in terms of contact hours, spent with child life specialists.

Results of this study demonstrated some change in parent report of child functioning, but there was not a difference in child report of their mental health symptoms between the two groups (Chernoff *et al.*, 2002). Although differences were small, parent report indicated fewer children who were not well adjusted in the intervention *versus* the comparison group. Dosage of the intervention and type of illness did not impact study findings. This may have occurred because the measures used for child report were designed to assess significant problems in depression and anxiety, and children did not exhibit large changes during the course of the study. Alternately, it may be that the children in the comparison group received sufficient support from the medical team and support of other mothers, which buffered them against stressors. Further study is needed to determine the impact of supportive interventions, especially for children and mothers who are not coping well with adjustment to the child's illness.

PARENT PERCEPTIONS IMPACT THE CHILD

Research indicating that parental perceptions of child vulnerability influence child perceptions of their own illness has yielded mixed results. For example, Mullins *et al.,* (2007) found that parental perceptions of child vulnerability were not related to child illness uncertainty in a group of children and adolescents with Type 1 Diabetes and asthma. Children may have been relatively well adjusted, which may have impacted study findings. However, parents with very high levels of stress were more likely to have children who reported higher levels of uncertainty. It may be that parent emotional functioning does play a role in child perceptions of the severity of his or her illness.

Anthony *et al.,* (2003) discovered a relationship between parental beliefs regarding child adjustment and children's ratings of their anxiety in social situations. They investigated the perceptions of sixty-nine parent-child dyads recruited from rheumatology and pulmonary clinics. They reported that parents with less education had higher perceptions of their child's vulnerability, related to increased levels of child worry. Anthony *et al.,* (2003) concluded that this may occur because parents with less education may be less likely to ask doctors about disease management. This idea was speculative in nature, and this is an area for future research.

In a large scale review paper, Cousino and Hazen (2013) reported that parent stress may be directly related to the burden they feel from caregiving and medical management of their child's illness. Parents perceiving a greater care-giving burden may be more stressed. Clinicians should assess parental coping and stress levels to determine when to provide counseling or make referrals.

Palermo and Eccleston (2009) discussed the impact of parent coping for children experiencing chronic pain. They proposed that parents can inadvertently influence a child's reactions to chronic pain. If parents of children experiencing chronic illnesses are depressed, anxious, and experience a significant amount of somatic symptoms, this can negatively impact their child's adjustment. Parent feelings of distress and upset may be highest in the first year post diagnosis, and this is a critical time for mental health providers to assess parent functioning and intervene to provide support and education to distressed parents (Palermo & Eccleston, 2009). Others have reported high levels of parent trauma in the first month or two after a child is injured or diagnosed with a chronic illness, with parent distress and trauma decreasing significantly over the course of the first year of coping with the stressor. Landolt *et al.*, (2012) found that maternal and paternal post-traumatic stress was much higher at five to six weeks post-diagnosis compared to these levels at a year post-diagnosis. We need to learn more about factors facilitating parent and child adjustment in the month after diagnosis. In addition, Palermo and Eccleston (2009) called for continued longitudinal study of parent factors and child adjustment.

Just as parent distress can have a negative impact (Palermo & Eccleston, 2009), the reverse is true, which is that positive parental behaviors and attitudes can positively impact child adjustment. Guion and Mrug (2012) assessed the role of parent and child adjustment in adolescents with cystic fibrosis and diabetes. Their findings suggested that parental optimism can have a positive, uplifting impact on adolescent functioning, resulting in fewer mental health problems for children with chronic medical conditions. Like Friedman *et al.*, (2004) and Palermo and Eccleston (2009), Guion and Mrug called for longitudinal research to examine the child and parent functioning over time to understand how the interplay of these factors impact child adjustment. In contrast, parent solicitation of pain responses can reinforce the "sick role" and feelings of helplessness in regard to disease management which may negatively impact child adjustment (Peterson & Palermo, 2004). In a similar vein, minimizing the child's adjustment and the serious nature of the illness or being negative about how the illness is affecting the family (*e.g.*, adopting a negative attitude about the child being ill) can negatively influence child adjustment and coping (Peterson & Palermo, 2004).

MULTIPLE FACTORS ASSOCIATED WITH PARENT FUNCTIONING INFLUENCE THE CHILD

Whittemore *et al.,* (2012) investigated parental functioning when one of their children had diabetes. They reviewed thirty-four articles that provided information about parent functioning. Their findings demonstrated that about 20-30% of parents were experiencing significant distress because their child had diabetes. Whittemore *et al.*, (2012) reported that more parents were likely to experience significant distress in the first year after their child received his or her diagnosis. However, they conducted a longitudinal study, and although distress decreased for many parents over a four-year interval, approximately 19% of parents exhibited stress at some point over the four years that study data were gathered. These researchers also indicated that 20-60% of the parents expressed symptoms of anxiety, while 10-74% reported depressive symptoms.

Friedman *et al.*, (2004) assessed the impact of several aspects of parent functioning on child adjustment, comparing the functioning of children with spina bifida to a group of children who were developing normally. Their findings suggested that paternal functioning and stress were related to child functioning for children with spina bifida. Although parents of children with spina bifida may experience greater stress, the processes through which parent stress, parent psychosocial functioning, and marital stress affect child functioning worked similarly in both groups.

The study by Friedman *et al.*, (2004) had several strengths. The study was longitudinal in nature and assessed functioning of both mothers and fathers. Interestingly, these researchers also tested the strength of association between three aspects of parent functioning and child functioning. The three parent-level variables were parenting stress, parent perceptions of marital satisfaction, and parent psychosocial functioning. It was hypothesized that the relations among parent stress and child functioning would be higher than those between parent psychosocial functioning and child adjustment. Lastly, it was hypothesized that marital satisfaction would have the relatively weakest association with child functioning. Hypotheses about strength of associations were not supported, indicating that all variables related to parental functioning were important to consider. These researchers concluded that parents of children with spina bifida may be resilient, although they function under a high level of stress, in part related to their child's chronic illness.

ADJUSTMENT OF MOTHERS AND FATHERS

Dewey and Crawford (2007) investigated mothers' and fathers' adjustment to child chronic illness. They compared adjustment and a host of other factors for mothers and fathers of children with chronic illnesses, life-threatening chronic illnesses, and healthy children. Diabetes and asthma were the chronic illnesses that were not life-threatening, while muscular dystrophy and cystic fibrosis were considered life-threatening illnesses. Their findings revealed that family cohesion was positively related to adjustment for mothers and fathers. However, other than this factor, the picture for mothers and fathers varied. In general mothers were more stressed and reported more adjustment problems than fathers did. This is consistent with other literature in the field, showing that mothers may experience higher levels of post-traumatic stress compared to fathers in the year after their child was diagnosed with a chronic illness or was recovering from an injury (Landolt *et al.*, 2012).

Dewey and Crawford (2007) discovered that mothers also valued social support as crucial to adjustment, whereas fathers' perceptions of stressful events for the family and their need for medical information were related to their adjustment. Specifically, fathers who perceived higher levels of family stress and negative family events as well as fathers who asked more medically related questions were less well-adjusted than fathers who reported lower levels of the aforementioned stressors. Fathers of children with life-threatening conditions (*i.e.*, cystic fibrosis and muscular dystrophy) did report lower social support compared to fathers of children in the healthy comparison group or fathers of children who had diabetes or asthma (*i.e.*, health conditions not classified as life-threatening). In terms of the big picture, both mothers and fathers of children with any of the chronic illnesses were as well adjusted as mothers and fathers of healthy children, which may mean that in many instances parents are coping in a positive manner and may be marked by resilient functioning.

Whittemore *et al.*, (2012) also found that mothers reported higher stress levels compared to fathers. Parents who were very stressed had more difficulty caring for their child, which could lead to more negative health outcomes related to adherence problems. Finally, children who had been diagnosed with diabetes for a longer period of time had parents who were more stressed than those with more recent diagnoses. Parents who were distressed often also used relatively "ineffective" parenting and discipline techniques, which can contribute to problems with the child's functioning. This could have occurred due to the worsening of their disease, poor disease management, or general "wear and tear" on parents who had worked hard to cope with a significant stressor for their child. Further research about how and why parents "wear out" or become disengaged from caring for the child's medical regimen is needed, in order to inform interventions to improve adherence for children with chronic illnesses. Parents did report enhanced support and emotional functioning if they felt they could easily be in contact with the medical team for questions. The mental health provider can ensure that channels of communication are open, so that the parent feels he or she can approach the medical team with questions.

ROLES FOR THE MENTAL HEALTH PROVIDER

For those parents who seek support or more information, the child mental health professional may serve as a liaison between the parents and the medical team, explaining family issues and psychosocial issues that the child is facing. The mental health professional also can serve as a conduit for relaying messages and information from the medical team to the parents, especially if relations between the doctor/medical team and the parents are strained or in cases where scheduling mismatches occur and group meetings are not possible to schedule.

Research points to the importance of monitoring family cohesion or functioning (*e.g.*, Dewey & Crawford, 2007). As one might expect, families that have poor functioning before the child's diagnosis may have more difficulty coping with illness-related stressors. Likewise, families that lack support or cohesion and do not exhibit positive relations among family members may have more difficulty adapting to a child's illness. Using a life events scale (that assesses negative and stressful life events) may allow for assessment of the impact of other life stresses, in addition to the child's illness, that may negatively impact parent and/or family functioning. Being alert to and assessing the impact of parent functioning, family functioning and child adjustment will provide critical data to inform the clinician of where to intervene to support the child and his or her family.

The degree to which the child's illness is perceived as disrupting family routines and activities may impact parent stress and perceptions of the burden of the child's illness. These perceptions, in turn, can influence the child's attitudes toward his or her illness. Sawyer *et al.*, (2004) examined children's health-related quality of life in a longitudinal study of functioning for children with cystic fibrosis, diabetes, and asthma. Their findings indicated that children perceived their quality of life to be lower if they felt they were not able to participate in family activities. The extent to which the clinician can help parents plan to involve the child with a chronic illness in daily family routines and activities may improve the child's adjustment to and attitude toward his or her chronic illness. Improving child involvement in family activities also can impact perceptions of family cohesion, which are related to parent adjustment (Dewey & Crawford, 2007). Over time, as the child and family adjust to coping with the child's illness, the mental health provider may experience less need to meet with and develop interventions for the family, as child involvement in the family, with peers, and at school can improve (Sawyer *et al.*, 2004). If this is the case, then the mental health professional can intervene "as needed" or in times of crisis and this "rubber band" approach – which involves being there when needed, and "hanging lose" during periods of family and child resilience may be a beneficial stance for the counselor.

Parents of children who have chronic illnesses may be overprotective of their child. It can be difficult to promote child involvement in disease management and child independence when parents view their child as being continually vulnerable due to his or her medical condition. Parents may experience difficulty allowing their child to become involved in independent activities if they feel that they need to continually monitor the child's health status. For children with chronic illnesses, attending a summer camp might be a first step in beginning to move toward some independence from parents and family. Once the child is successful at a camp, a next step may be increase child involvement in extra-curricular activities, with advice and guidance from the medical team being provided to adults leading these activities.

If a parent is being overprotective, the mental health provider needs to process this issue with the parent. One way to address this issue is to discuss it as a normal reaction that is not helpful for the child's long-term independence and development. Parental overprotection could be explained as a normal reaction that has intensified or is prolonged due to concern for the child. Although it has a positive foundation, when carried to an extreme level it can limit the child. As this notion is reviewed the clinician can work with the parent(s) to develop a more realistic picture of what their child can and cannot accomplish independently. In order to develop a realistic picture of the child's abilities, the mental health provider may need to arrange meetings with the medical team so that these experts can provide factual information about the child's physical, intellectual and psychosocial skills as well as about the level of support and scaffolding that will be necessary for the child to improve his or her involvement in age-appropriate activities.

One possible intervention is to assist a parent in making contact with another parent with a child facing similar issues (Chernoff *et al.*, 2002). Another way to help a parent reach out is to refer the parent to local, state, or national support groups for children with similar health problems. Or, connecting the parent with another parent who also visits the medical team can be helpful, provided parents in both parties provide consent to be introduced to one another. Another strategy is to encourage the parent to ask a member of the medical team, such as the nurse or attending physician, to find a "peer mentor." This experienced parent can share ideas for management of the child's symptoms. Asking questions about caregiver or parent perceptions of stress and burden for their child's medical care will provide background information to determine whether the parent needs counseling support to cope with their child's medical condition (Cousino & Hazen, 2013).

Parent and child grief reactions to the stress of the illness may be common, especially in the first year following a new diagnosis (Landolt *et al.*, 2012; Palermo & Eccleston, 2009). As such, mental health providers should gain expertise in counseling related to grief and loss issues. Attending workshops and seminars in this area can provide a wealth of experience for clinicians. Reviewing books and articles presenting information on interventions to promote positive coping and adjustment to grief may provide helpful guidance, and therefore a list of such references in presented in Table **1**.

A percentage of parents may experience significant distress related to their child's chronic illness. The mental health provider working with children needs to ensure that he or she has appropriate skills for identifying parents who are having significant difficulty coping with grief related to their child's illness or who are experiencing depression and anxiety secondary to accepting and coping with their child's medical condition.

Table 1:   References for Coping with Trauma and Grief

Hooyman, N. R., & Kramer, B. J. (2006). *Living through loss: Interventions across the life span*. New York: Columbia University Press.
Humphrey, K. M. (2009). *Counseling strategies for loss and grief*. Alexandria, VA: American Counseling Association.
Litz, B. T. (Ed.). (2004). *Early intervention for trauma and traumatic loss*. New York: Guilford Press.
Stroebe, M. S., Hansson, R. O., Schut, H., & Stroebe, W. (Eds). (2008). *Handbook of bereavement research and practice: Advances in theory and intervention*. Washington, D.C.: American Psychological Association.
Worden, J. W. (2009). *Grief counseling and grief therapy: A handbook for the mental health practitioner, Fourth Edition*. New York: Springer Publishing.

Single parents may be at high risk for experiencing stress, anxiety and/or depression when their child has a chronic illness. A work group of pediatric psychologists reviewed the literature and found that single parents are likely to experience financial stress, anxiety related to adjusting to the medical system and family separation, and worry about their child (Brown *et al.*, 2008). Single parents may be particularly stressed, because they do not have the resources to both attend to the child with the illness and take care of other siblings in the family. Brown and his colleagues concluded that research adding information about the functioning of single parents will provide information for interventions. Mental health providers should be aware of this issue and how to provide support for single parents in terms of both counseling support and assistance with other types of instrumental support, such as child care, transportation, *etc.*

CASE STUDY: GIRL WITH SICKLE CELL ANEMIA

This case study presents information for assessment and counseling of a single parent. Rebecca was a single parent, with three young children under the age of 10 years. Her middle child, Krissa, has been diagnosed with sickle cell anemia. Krissa has been in and out of the hospital battling a series of infections. Rebecca is struggling with the fact that she is a carrier for this trait. She is tired and worried about her ability to manage her full-time work, her other two children's care and schedules, and Krissa's medical appointments. Krissa also has had emergency room visits for pain related to vaso-occlusive crises. During these crises she was given morphine and Rebecca worries that this drug is "addicting" and may have long-term consequences for Krissa. When thinking about Krissa's adult years, Rebecca worries about other complications that may occur in those with sickle cell disease, such as problems with breathing (acute chest syndrome), sickle retinopathy, and pain in her bones -- with possible loss of spleen functioning.

Over time, Rebecca has restricted her social circle to only immediate family members. She no longer does anything in terms of her own self-care. She has recently lost 10 pounds and never feels like eating. She has difficulty sleeping through the night. Her two children who are developing typically and are "healthy" complain that she does not have enough time to spend with them. Rebecca is fiercely protective of Krissa, immediately responding with kisses, treats, and candy when Krissa reports feeling "pain in my legs and arms." Rebecca frequently does not allow Krissa to play outside for fear she will be exposed to germs and suffer from another round of pneumonia, the most common infection she has incurred since being diagnosed with sickle cell anemia. Rebecca feels responsible for her daughter's chronic illness and is guilt-ridden over her daughter's missed childhood opportunities. The symptoms of sadness are not severe and have been occurring for the past 4 months or so. This recent difficulty adjusting to her daughter's condition came after worrying that her insurance for her daughter, in terms of covering her daughter's health care, would "run out." Rebecca's job, in a local pizzeria, would not provide enough funds to cover the expenses related to sickle cell disease.

The attending physician caring for Krissa had recently noticed a change in Rebecca's demeanor. Rebecca had expressed some of her worries about caring for her daughter and the other children in the family to Krissa's physician. Rebecca, a single parent, has some support from her parents and older sister, but faces a substantial care-giving burden. In light of this, the attending physician thought it prudent to refer Rebecca for a visit with a social worker at the children's hospital.

Rebecca made her first contact with the social worker at one of Krissa's clinic visits – a monthly check-up after her recent discharge from the hospital due to a bout of pneumonia and pain crises related to her sickle cell anemia. The attending physician approached Rebecca about the possibility of speaking with the social worker and she agreed to meet her at one of Krissa's regularly scheduled clinic appointments. She did not feel she had the time or resources to set a separate appointment to meet with the social worker, as she has already missed significant time at work, resulting in monetary losses. The social worker, Ms. Pam, was introduced by the attending physician. The conversation between Rebecca and Ms. Pam began with Ms. Pam explaining her role at the children's hospital. Rebecca appeared to establish rapport and an alliance with Ms. Pam. Because of this, Ms. Pam felt comfortable asking Rebecca to talk about ways in which Krissa and the family needed support. This indirect approach allowed Rebecca to begin to talk about family issues, without a direct focus on her needs, which have always taken a "back seat" to the needs of her children.

Rebecca mentioned that she was terribly worried about her insurance benefits for Krissa and the other children "running out." She reported that this concern is, "Keeping me up at night." Ms. Pam asked Rebecca if she was aware of the State Children's Health Insurance Plan or SCHIP. This program, designed to provide health care coverage to children residing in low-income families living in the United States, provides independent insurance for children who need their own insurance coverage. Rebecca had not realized that there was such a program and that all three of her children would be eligible for care under SCHIP. She agreed to meet with Ms. Pam to fill out paperwork at Krissa's next visit.

At Krissa's next clinic visit, Ms. Pam and Rebecca talked more about Krissa's illness and Rebecca's concerns for her daughter's current medical care and her concerns about possible long-term health consequences related to sickle cell anemia. At this conversation progressed, Rebecca mentioned how important faith is to her and how she misses opportunities to participate in Church. Since recently moving to be nearer to the children's hospital, Rebecca has not found a local church for her and her family. Ms. Pam asked if she could locate a nearby church and bring Rebecca information about the church at the next clinic visit. Rebecca hesitantly agreed to this plan.

Soon, the next visit arrived. Ms. Pam was scheduled to meet with Rebecca at the end of the clinic visit. During the visit, a child life specialist spent time playing with Krissa. Ms. Pam provided Rebecca with information on two local churches with strong youth programs. Ms. Pam brought contact information and telephone numbers for a church member and the pastor at each church. After this exchange of information, Ms. Pam showed SCHIP paperwork to Rebecca. Together they worked to complete the paperwork. Rebecca commented, "I feel better...I just wish there was something to lift me up too." Ms. Pam replies, "Lift you up?" Rebecca answers, "Yes, make me feel supported and give me a break." Ms. Pam inquires if by getting a break Rebecca needs respite care for her daughter, a vacation, or support for herself. Rebecca clarified that she needed mentoring to discuss how to care for Krissa when she experiences pain. She stated that she would like to talk with another mother who knows what it is like to "go through hospital visits and stays due to sickle cell pain."

Ms. Pam asked Rebecca if she was familiar with the mothers' support group for children with sickle cell anemia. Rebecca replied that she had not known such a group existed. Rebecca asked if she could have some names and telephone numbers to contact a few mothers in the group. Ms. Pam went back to her office and found some contact information. She also returned with a flier showing dates and times for monthly meetings of the "Mothers of Children with Sickle Cell Support Group." Ms. Pam informed Rebecca that child life specialists were available at the monthly meetings to provide child care, so that children were welcome to accompany their parents to the group. Rebecca reported that she was relieved to hear about this because she did not often have child care or babysitters. Ms. Pam stated that mothers in the group would be a good source for finding child care and that sometimes they "traded" babysitting.

At the next visit, Rebecca reported she had found a church home. She said that she had contacted, "a person at the Mothers' Support Group so that I can attend the next monthly meeting." She was still hesitant about contacting individual mothers to ask for mentoring. Ms. Pam praised her efforts at coping and let Rebecca know that the paperwork for SCHIP was submitted and they were waiting for a response. Rebecca then talked a bit about herself. She explained to Ms. Pam that since her daughter's last hospitalization and concerns about her insurance not covering her daughter's care she had become sad. Rebecca admitted that she was not sleeping through the night and was skipping meals and losing weight. Ms. Pam asked Rebecca to rate her sad feelings on a scale from "one to ten, with 10 being very sad." Rebecca said that most days she was at "two or three, but when Krissa is in the hospital I'm at a five sometimes." Ms. Pam asked Rebecca how long these feelings had been going on and she said, "About two months or so." Ms. Pam told Rebecca she might be having an adjustment reaction to recent stresses and asked if Rebecca would like to talk to someone about her concerns.

After a few moments of reflection, Rebecca mentioned that she would like to try counseling. Ms. Pam asked if she could run back to her office and find referral information. Ms. Pam returned shortly with the names of three counselors who either accepted Rebecca's insurance or worked on a sliding scale in terms of charging for services. Ms. Pam also returned with the name of one mother she thought might be a good mentor for Rebecca, as her daughter had been coping with sickle cell anemia for twelve years. Rebecca happily reported she felt comfortable contacting one mother for mentoring. Rebecca said she might call one of the counselors, but stated that although she needed counseling she was not sure if she had the time, desire, or energy to seek her own mental health services. Ms. Pam thought about this and asked if the stigma related to seeking mental health services was limiting Rebecca's avenues for support. Rebecca indicated that this was the case, and then Ms. Pam asked about possible referral for counseling sessions with the Pastor at Rebecca's church. Rebecca felt positively about this idea and also wanted to join a Bible study group.

At her next visit, Rebecca started the meeting by thanking Ms. Pam for her support and the referral information. Rebecca had joined a local Bible study group and had met a friend there. She said that attending this group was the highlight of her week. She had met one time with Pastor Joe and thought she had greatly benefitted from discussing her problems with him. Ms. Pam asked about Rebecca's sadness and worry on a scale of one to ten (again). Rebecca happily reported that she was usually at a "level two, but this is just mostly when I worry about my kids." Rebecca was feeling much better, and was now sleeping and eating regularly.

Rebecca had attended a monthly support group for Mothers of Children with Sickle Cell Anemia and had a wonderful time. At this group she met with the "mentor" Ms. Pam had suggested. This mother was contacting her one time per week to offer support and to provide advice. Rebecca believed this support was a, "lifeline, giving me insight into the future and how to do the best for my daughter, Krissa." Rebecca mentioned that she was doing much better and would like to keep Ms. Pam's card in case she needed to speak with her again. Ms. Pam readily agreed to this plan.

Ms. Pam mentioned that Krissa might benefit from a visit from the pediatric psychologist consulting with the sickle cell team at her next clinic visit. An appointment was set with Dr. Brinkmeyer, a pediatric psychologist with expertise in pain management. During the first meeting rapport was established. Rebecca also provided background information about Krissa's pain coping and her role in helping Krissa cope with pain. Rebecca felt comfortable with Dr. Brinkmeyer and let her know that she wanted her daughter to be fully protected from any negative experiences or exposure to any germs at school. Dr. Brinkmeyer was able to process with Rebecca that if this occurred, Krissa would be limited, in terms of social interactions and chances to make friends and develop her social skills. Rebecca had not thought of this, and in ongoing sessions with Dr. Brinkmeyer Rebecca was able to discuss her worries for her child. She became open to talking about and eventually understanding how her overprotection of Krissa was limiting her social development.

Dr. Brinkmeyer and Rebecca talked about how some of Rebecca's behaviors might be accidentally "rewarding" Krissa's pain complaints. For example, Dr. Brinkmeyer discussed how rewarding pain complaints with candy might inadvertently reinforce and therefore increase pain complaints. Dr. Brinkmeyer educated Rebecca about relaxation and distraction as pain control strategies. As a team, Dr. Brinkmeyer and Rebecca worked to teach Krissa to use mental imagery to relax, by thinking of attending her birthday party or thinking about a visit to a local amusement park. They talked about the importance of doing fun things in order to help Krissa take her mind off her pain and focus on something she enjoyed doing. Rebecca and Dr. Brinkmeyer developed a reward chart and Krissa began to receive rewards (*e.g.*, playing a game with her mother) for practicing her pain management strategies.

In time, Krissa's pain reports decreased and Krissa began to let her mother know that, "I can deal with my pain by myself with my strategies sometimes." At times multiple strategies were used, including distraction and relaxation as well as using warm towels and drinking lots of water when Krissa had "pain in my bones." Krissa became more outgoing and soon developed a best friend at school. She began to sing in the choir at her church, which was an activity that boosted her self-esteem. After two months had passed, Krissa reported higher feelings of self-efficacy for being able to "do what I need to do to take care of my pain." Krissa stated that, "I can work on my pain on my own and I do not always need to tell Mommy."

CONCLUSION

This chapter reviewed issues for parents of children with chronic illness. Parental support and ideas for working with the child may be gained from professionals or peer mentors who have children facing similar medical issues. Support can be gained from multiple professional and nonprofessional avenues. Time to establish rapport and learn about how to fit supports with parental values and family lifestyle are crucial ingredients to developing a plan for helping the parent. Supporting the child, by teaching pain management or disease management strategies or finding counseling for the child may be a key ingredient in empowering parents.

Ideas for supporting the parent include finding peer mentors, counseling referrals, and improving parent involvement in extracurricular activities so that the parent has more opportunities to engage in self-care. A rationale for empowering the parent may be found in this analogy – think about being on a plane in an emergency. If the air masks fall, then the parent needs to breathe in the mask before placing it on their child's nose and mouth. Thus, with a little self-care the parent gains abilities to better care for his or her child. The notion of taking care of yourself so that you can help and support your child "more" may provide parents with the permission they may need to attend to the self and reduce their guilt and feelings of depression and anxiety. The case example at the end of this chapter focused on a mother who was exhibiting relatively mild feelings of depression, grief over her child's condition, and anxiety. The mental health professional should be well-versed in assessment of adult functioning so that he or she can provide appropriate referral for parent services as needed. Consequently, in order to provide good services, the mental health provider needs to be well-trained to assess parent functioning, knowledgeable about support services in the community, and knowledgeable about strategies for managing the child's chronic illness.

ACKNOWLEDGEMENTS

None declared.

CONFLICT OF INTEREST

The author confirms that this chapter contents have no conflict of interest.

REFERENCES

Anthony, K. K., Gil, K. M., & Schanberg, L. E. (2003). Brief report: Parental perceptions of child vulnerability in children with chronic illness. *Journal of Pediatric Psychology, 28*(3), 185-190.

Brown, R. T., Wiener, L., Kupst, M. J., Brennan, T., Behrman, R., Compas, B. *et al.* (2008). Single parents of children with chronic illness: An understudied phenomenon. *Journal of Pediatric Psychology, 33*(4), 408-421.

Chernoff, R. G., Ireys, H. T., Devet, K. A., & Kim, Y. J. (2002). A randomized controlled trial of a community-based support program for families of children with chronic illness: Pediatric outcomes. *Archives of Pediatrics and Adolescent Medicine, 156*(6), 533-539.

Coffey, J. S. (2006). Parenting a child with a chronic illness: A metasynthesis. *Pediatric Nursing, 32*, 51-59.

Cousino, M. K., & Hazen, R. A. (2013). Parenting stress among caregivers of children with chronic illness: A systematic review. *Journal of Pediatric Psychology, 38*(8), 809-828.

Dewey, D., & Crawford, S. G. (2007). Correlates of maternal and paternal adjustment to chronic childhood disease. *Journal of Clinical Psychology in Medical Settings, 14*, 219-226.

Friedman, D., Holmbeck, G. N., Jandasak, B., Zuckerman, J., & Abad, M. (2004). Parent functioning in families of preadolescents with spina bifida: Longitudinal implications of child adjustment. *Journal of Family Psychology, 18*(4), 609-617.

Guion, K., & Mrug, S. (2012). The role of parental and adolescent attribution in adjustment of adolescents with chronic illness. *Journal of Clinical Psychology in Medical Settings, 19*(3), 262-269.

Hooyman, N. R., & Kramer, B. J. (2006). *Living through loss: Interventions across the life span.* New York: Columbia University Press.

Humphrey, K. M. (2009). *Counseling strategies for loss and grief.* Alexandria, VA: American Counseling Association.

Landolt, M. A., Ystrom, E., Sennhausen, F. H., Gnehm, H. E., & Vollrath, M. E. (2012). The mutual prospective influence of child and parental post-traumatic stress symptoms in pediatric patients. *Journal of Child Psychology and Psychiatry, 53*(7), 767-774.

Litz, B. T. (Ed.). (2004). *Early intervention for trauma and traumatic loss.* New York: Guilford Press.

Mullins, L. L., Wolfe-Christensen, C., Hoff-Pai, A. L., Carpentier, M. Y., Gillapsy, S., Check, J., & Page, M. (2007). The relationship of parental overprotection, perceived child vulnerability, and parenting stress to uncertainty in youth with chronic illness. *Journal of Pediatric Psychology, 32*(8), 973-982.

Palermo, T. M., & Eccleston, C. (2009). Parents of children and adolescents with chronic pain. *Pain, 146*(1-2), 15-17.

Peterson, C. C., & Palermo, T. M. (2004). Parental reinforcement of recurrent pain: The moderating impact of child depression and anxiety on functional disability. *Journal of Pediatric Psychology, 29*(5), 331-341.

Sawyer, M. G., Reynolds, K. E., Couper, J. J., French, D. J., Kennedy, D., Martin, J. *et al.* (2004). Health-related quality of life of children and adolescents with chronic illness—a two year prospective study. *Quality of Life Research, 13*, 1309-1319.

Stroebe, M. S., Hansson, R. O., Schut, H., & Stroebe, W. (Eds). (2008). *Handbook of bereavement research and practice: Advances in theory and intervention.* Washington, D.C.: American Psychological Association.

Whittemore, R., Jaser, S., Chao, A., Jang, M., & Grey, M. (2012). Psychological experience of parents of children with Type 1 Diabetes: A systematic mixed studies review. *Diabetes Educator, 38*(4), 562-579.

Worden, J. W. (2009). *Grief counseling and grief therapy: A handbook for the mental health practitioner, Fourth Edition.* New York: Springer Publishing.

CHAPTER 8

Adjustment of Siblings of Children with Chronic Illnesses

Laura A. Nabors[*]

Health Education Program, School of Human Services, University of Cincinnati, 468 Dyer Hall, Mail Location 0068, Cincinnati, Ohio, OH 45221-0068, USA

Abstract: Siblings of children who have chronic medical conditions can experience both positive and negative outcomes related to their brother or sister's illness. For example, siblings can experience increased empathy and compassion. Their bonds with their brother or sister typically are affectionate. The downside is that siblings can feel isolated and "in need" of parental attention. Improving support from parents, school staff, and peers, as well as allowing siblings to express their feelings are positive techniques for improving their coping. Interventions to educate and support siblings appear to have a beneficial impact on sibling functioning and remain an area for future research.

Keywords: Sibling adjustment, sibling coping, siblings' grief, sibling isolation, supporting siblings.

INTRODUCTION

Siblings of children with chronic illnesses experience a myriad of feelings and reactions to a brother or sister's chronic illness. Besier *et al.,* (2010) found that approximately one-third of siblings of children with chronic illness exhibited some issues with emotional and behavioral functioning. Siblings may suffer from stress, sadness, and anxiety over the course of their brother or sister's chronic illness (Alderfer *et al.,* 2003). They also can experience feelings of guilt over their own positive health (Gilmore *et al.*, 2012; Redshaw & Wilson, 2012). They may feel left out or lonely and long for parental attention (Lemarche & Newton, 2012). Some children may have difficulty understanding the illness and its treatment (Gilmore *et al.*, 2012). Siblings are at risk for suppressing their feelings, so as not

---

*Address correspondence to **Laura A. Nabors:** Health Education Program, School of Human Services, University of Cincinnati, 468 Dyer Hall, Mail Location 0068, Cincinnati, Ohio, OH 45221-0068, USA; Tel: 513-556-5537; Fax: 513-556-3898; E-mail: naborsla@ucmail.uc.edu

to bother their parents, which can lead to problems with their emotional functioning (Vermaes *et al.,* 2012).

Menke (1987) completed interviews with seventy-two siblings, between six and twelve years of age, and their parents. She concluded that siblings and parents did agree that siblings expressed concern over their brother or sister's welfare. Siblings reported that parents were often busy with caring for their brother or sister, were worried, and could be very tired. Approximately one-third of the siblings reported that they helped out and behaved better at home since their brother or sister was ill. About a quarter of the sample reported that they were receiving more support from teachers or extended family associated with their brother or sister's illness. Many parents thought that the siblings were well-adjusted and that their school performance had remained steady. Menke documented some positive impact on sibling functioning as they strove to cope with their brother or sister's illness and assist their parents. Menke *et al.,* (2009) mentioned that both positive and negative sibling adjustment is possible. They suggested understanding the child's behavior and "contentment" with life in order to understand sibling adjustment when a brother or sister is facing a chronic illness.

Williams *et al.,* (2009) assessed parent perceptions of the effects of a brother or sister's chronic illness on sibling functioning. The brother or sister had either cancer or cystic fibrosis. These illnesses were selected because they can be life-threatening and have a significant impact on family functioning. Forty-four parents were interviewed – 29 had children who had cancer and 15 had a child coping with cystic fibrosis. Mothers were the typical respondents – and it is noteworthy that more information is needed about fathers' perceptions of sibling functioning. Williams *et al.,* (2009) reported five themes in parent responses including, "jealous/envious; worry/fear/anxiety; upset/anger/resentment; lonely/sad/depressed; other negative behaviors; and other problems (such as school problems)." (p. 100). When one reviews the five themes, another plausible interpretation is that more themes were evident, because some of the themes appeared "lumped" together. For example, feelings of loneliness and sadness may be two different types of emotional reactions. Parent perceptions of sibling adaptation appeared more negative – in comparison to the findings reported by

Menke (1987). This may have occurred because the children with illnesses were facing life-threatening conditions and this may evoke different reactions in siblings. Therefore, in studies with larger samples, it will be important to compare the functioning of siblings with brothers or sisters with life-threatening illnesses *versus* siblings of children with illnesses that are not considered life-threatening.

Waite-Jones and Madill (2008) discussed the reactions and adjustment of siblings of children with juvenile idiopathic arthritis. Their findings showed that siblings experience some ambivalence related to their brother or sister's conditions. There were positive findings, since siblings often,

"...displayed a strong sense of what being a good brother or sister should be. They acted as advocates and protectors... (p. 486).

Another possible positive outcome was that the family could become closer as they pulled together to battle their brother or sister's chronic illness. Ambivalence or less positive feelings could occur if the sibling felt a loss of time spent with peers and parents or a loss of parental attention. Some siblings expressed that a brother or sister could exaggerate or amplify symptoms related to arthritis for attention and other secondary gains, such as not having to go to school or complete chores at home. Hence, it appeared that there could be positive and negative outcomes for siblings when a brother or sister had juvenile idiopathic arthritis.

Siblings can gain perspectives in new areas that are positive for their emotional growth. For instance, they may gain insights that improve their compassion and empathy for others experiencing personal difficulties or hardships (Gilmore *et al.*, 2012). They may become more mature, and become more independent and able to care for themselves (Redshaw & Wilson, 2012). Hence, siblings may experience a mix of positive and negative feelings, and above all, feel love and feelings of care for their brother or sister (Hames & Appleton, 2009).

Vermaes *et al.,* (2012) conducted a meta-analysis to examine psychological functioning of siblings. They reviewed fifty-two studies and their results indicated that siblings may face emotional problems and have less positive self-perceptions.

Siblings may suppress any feelings that they may have, leading to internalizing problems, because they do not want to burden their parents. Internalizing problems, such as sadness and anxiety, may be more prevalent than "acting out" or externalizing problems. In terms of having difficulty with positive perceptions of personal attributes, findings indicated that older siblings may have more difficulty with positive self-perceptions. Moreover, siblings of children with life-threatening chronic illnesses may experience more emotional difficulties. Additionally, siblings in very large families may experience less parental support and have more adjustment difficulties (O'Brien *et al.*, 2009). Vermaes *et al.*, (2012) believed that further research will be needed to determine how the interaction between the parent and the sibling influences family dynamics and sibling functioning.

ENHANCING SIBLING KNOWLEDGE AND INVOLVEMENT IN FAMILY COPING

O'Haver *et al.*, (2010) assessed parent perceptions of risk and protective factors for the adjustment of siblings of youngsters with cystic fibrosis. Parents of 40 siblings of children with cystic fibrosis provided information on behavioral and emotional functioning, social support, stress, and severity of the brother or sister's illness. Results demonstrated that parent stress and lack of parent social support were risk factors for poor adjustment of siblings. Children residing in low-income families could have poorer adjustment. Consequently, one might assume that supporting parents and reducing parental stress would have an indirect and positive impact on sibling functioning. Additionally, screening siblings in families with lower resources, such as those with less financial support, for stress is an important consideration.

O'Haver *et al.*, (2010) found that siblings could exhibit internalizing problems, such as depression or anxiety. Younger siblings had more adjustment problems compared to adolescents. This could have occurred because younger siblings perceived their burden of care to be more stressful. This idea is speculative. It is based on research by O'Brien *et al.*, (2009) who reported that siblings who perceive their caregiving burden as being heavy and their parent support as relatively low could be at risk for exhibiting behavioral problems.

O'Haver *et al.*, (2010) noted that "...75% of the well siblings had never spoken to the medical team about their brother or sister's illness (p. 290). O'Haver *et al.*, (2010) believed that siblings could benefit from the educational information and support they could receive from the medical team. Conversations with team members could improve their knowledge and offer them a source of support. Siblings who exhibited poor emotional and behavioral functioning prior to diagnosis of the chronic illness for their brother or sister, tended to be at risk for poor adjustment after the diagnosis. These researchers added that siblings may have even more concerns for a brother or sister and need even more support as their brother or sister ages and deals with increasing disease symptomatology. They called for provision of more resources and education for families of children with cystic fibrosis and this is a call that could be helpful for families of children with a myriad of chronic illnesses, in terms of increasing support for siblings and parents and buffering both against stress.

Another way to help siblings is to set aside time to interact with them and answer their questions. During this time, parents or caregivers have opportunities to teach the sibling about the illness. Another tip for assisting siblings is to teach them how to explain illness to other children, so that they are able to answer questions posed by peers (Gilmore *et al.*, 2012). When new family routines are built to adjust to illness, finding roles for siblings helps them find a place in the family. Gilmore *et al.*, (2012) suggested that caregivers should allow siblings to express their feelings about their brother or sister's illness – and they should be prepared for the sibling to wrestle with contrasting feelings, such as feeling very protective of their brother or sister, while at the same time feeling jealous that their brother or sister is getting "all" of the parents' attention. When appropriate, such as when sibling adjustment is compromised and they exhibit significant sadness and anxiety or behavior problems, then referral to a mental health care provider should be considered.

Lemarche and Newton (2012) suggested that sibling and parent involvement are intertwined and this was consistent with recommendations by Vermaes *et al.*, (2012) to direct further study toward increasing knowledge about how parent-child interaction impacts the adjustment of siblings of children with chronic health conditions. Lemarche and Newton added to this notion by indicating that parents should be involved in interventions to improve sibling functioning and further research examining the family, parent, and sibling adjustment may provide insights that shed light on the dynamic interactions that shape family development as a child copes with a chronic illness. Because siblings need education and information about their brother or sister's illness, parents may be the optimal persons to educate so that they can provide their children with this knowledge (Hames & Appleton, 2009).

Other researchers have found that positive family functioning is a buffer for siblings of children with chronic illnesses. Gold *et al.*, (2011) assessed how family support and conflict affected the functioning of 54 siblings of children who had sickle cell anemia. Their data "source" was a primary caregiver who provided information on one sibling in the family who was between eight and sixteen years of age. Gold *et al.*, (2011) found that sibling functioning was more positive when family support was higher and conflict within the family was relatively lower. They discovered that siblings of children with illnesses who had a higher number of emergency room visits were functioning poorer and showing less adjustment. This could occur because the children with illnesses that were more severe visited the emergency room more often.

Alternately, it could be that families of children with illnesses who attend the emergency room more often have a "last-minute" or "crisis" orientation to coping with illness, which has a less positive prognosis for sibling functioning. Gold *et al.,* (2011) stressed that clinicians need to assess sibling functioning as part of their assessment of the child with an illness and his or her family. Further research examining the role of interventions for siblings, such as participation in support groups or learning about their brother or sister's illness and how to cope with it through videos may be helpful. Or, if the siblings reside in a rural area or are removed from other families coping with the same situations, telehealth or videoconferencing might be a good method for providing education and support to siblings.

INTERVENTIONS TO IMPROVE SIBLING ADJUSTMENT

Redshaw and Wilson (2012) used interviews to evaluate family perceptions of a bead program on sibling involvement in the care of a child with a chronic heart disease. Qualitative methods were used to find themes in the interview data. The beads were provided by the hospital to document the story or journey the child with a heart condition faced. They found that involvement in making strings of beads and learning stories about the beads helped siblings understand what was happening to their brother or sister and at the same time involved them in the family narrative as the family adjusted to the brother or sister's chronic illness. Thus, the beads, "told the story" of the child's treatment and the beads were a teaching tool to explain the illness and treatment process to siblings. Redshaw and Wilson concluded that projects that involved and educated siblings, such as the bead program, could help siblings understand what was going on and be a part of the developing family story.

Lobato and Kao (2002) conducted a sibling and parent group intervention to improve sibling adjustment to a brother or sister's chronic illness or disability. They recruited 54 well siblings and their parents – a child in the family had either a chronic illness or a developmental disability – to participate in groups where the goal was to improve sibling knowledge of the illness or developmental disability, improve connection between the sibling and his or her brother or sister, and enhance perspective-taking skills. Their intervention was comprised of six 90-minute groups conducted over six to eight weeks. Sessions targeted managing emotions, problem-solving around difficult family situations, learning about a brother or sister's illness, and improving exchange of information and connectedness in the family. Siblings and parents participated in different groups. Sibling groups were led by doctoral students in psychology and the parent groups were run by a licensed psychologist. Siblings also created a videotape about their experience that parents reviewed to enhance their understanding of sibling experiences.

Labato and Kao (2002) found that sibling knowledge of their brother or sister's condition improved as did feelings of connectedness with the brother or sister. Concomitantly, parent report indicated improved sibling adjustment and decreased behavioral problems post-intervention. Parents had learned reasons for and ideas for problem-solving around sibling behavior, which may have positively influenced reductions in behavioral problems. Interestingly, siblings of children with developmental disabilities (such as autism) expressed less knowledge of their brother or sister's condition prior to participating in the groups and they may require additional information and explanation to gain a better understanding of the problems their brother or sister is experiencing. This study did not have a comparison group, and this limited the generalizability of study findings. Furthermore, the authors reported that they did not examine the interplay of sibling and parent behaviors and interactions, which would be critical to examine in future studies.

Besier *et al.*, (2010) assessed sibling adjustment after parents and siblings participated in an intervention to improve family functioning. Children were siblings of a brother or sister with cystic fibrosis, congenital heart disease, or cancer. Siblings participated in sessions to improve their understanding of their brother or sister's illness, teach them relaxation and ways to cope with their changing lives, and they participated in counseling sessions to support them in expressing their emotions. Sessions were held with parents and a focus was to strengthen the sibling-parent relationship. The emotional and behavior functioning of the siblings improved after the intervention and stayed improved at a six-month follow-up. There were no differences in sibling functioning based on type of illness for the brother or sister. Besier *et al.*, (2010) found that as emotional and behavioral problems decreased sibling reports of quality of life were elevated. Therefore, interventions to improve family functioning, sibling functioning, and parent-child relationships can be uplifting for a sibling, leading to improvements in functioning and life satisfaction. Given the relative dearth of research in this area, further study of interventions to identify siblings in need of intervention and developing interventions to support them and promote their functioning is needed.

USE MULTIPLE SOURCES OF INFORMATION TO ASSESS SIBLING FUNCTIONING

It is advisable to use multiple sources of information to learn about sibling functioning. Parents are good sources of information as are informal observations of family functioning. When learning about the family one question to ask is, "how are siblings adjusting to _____ (name of child with illness) medical condition?" Follow-up questions can assess sibling emotional and behavioral functioning, participation in family activities, relationships with caregivers, and social development. Different family members may have different perceptions of sibling functioning. Observations, to confirm reports about sibling functioning, can provide useful information for the clinician. Reports about sibling functioning at school and with peers (in social situations) can provide other useful information.

Neilson *et al.,* (2011) reported that mothers and fathers may have differing perceptions of sibling functioning when a brother or sister in the family is coping with a chronic illness. These researchers investigated parental perceptions across various illness types. They discovered that mothers rated siblings as being more empathic than fathers did. Mothers also reported that older siblings might be more likely to avoid interactions with a brother or sister who had a chronic illness. In contrast, fathers saw differences in sibling coping based on the type of illness or disability that their brother or sister was coping with. Fathers believed that siblings of children with autism or with Down syndrome displayed more kindness to their brother or sister than siblings of children with either diabetes or orthopedic conditions. Hence, type of illness for the child with the chronic illness may effect siblings' reactions toward the illness and their interactions with their brother or sister. This study relied on reports of parents and adding observational data might have strengthened study findings, if observations were consistent with mothers' and/or fathers' reports.

Menke (1987) included the questions she asked parents and siblings. She asked siblings what they knew of their brother or sister's condition, who told them, if their lives had changed since their brother or sister became ill, what it was like for them when their brother or sister was in the hospital, what they worried about, what they might like to talk about with a brother or sister with an illness, and whether they had someone to speak with about their worries. Menke also asked the siblings to describe what was difficult about having a brother or sister who was ill and whether their lives had changed due to their brother or sister's condition. Parents provided information about the sibling's school and behavioral functioning and whether they had increased somatic complaints. Parents also provided information about siblings' interactions with peers and their perceptions of whether the sibling was coping with a lot of worries related to a brother or sister's illness. These questions seemed practical and a guide for those assessing parent and sibling perceptions of the adjustment of siblings who have a brother or sister coping with a chronic illness.

As mentioned, Williams *et al.*, (2009) assessed parent perceptions of sibling functioning when a brother or sister had a life-threatening chronic illness. One of the quotes in the article was striking. One mother stated that the sibling felt that the parent loved the ill child more than her. If this occurs, it would be important for the parent and sibling to talk and spend time together to ensure that the sibling's feelings of self-worth are supported. Spending quality time with a caregiver – or another extended family member – can support a sibling if he or she is feeling "left-out" in terms of receiving adult attention. It seems that parents and other members of the medical team need to assess sibling functioning, especially in terms of feelings of belongingness, when checking on sibling adjustment. Another potential source of information about sibling functioning is to assess their friendships and other peer relationships in order to determine if their social supports and peer interactions are positive and fulfilling in nature (O'Brien *et al.*, 2009).

INCREASING COMMUNICATION AND PROVIDING SCHOOL SUPPORT

Improving family communication is one avenue for facilitating sibling coping and adjustment when a brother or sister is suffering from a chronic illness. Herzer *et al.*, (2010) discovered that communication among family members was unclear in approximately 25% of families who had a child suffering from a chronic illness. Additionally, about one-third of the families had problems with affective involvement in the family. Consequently, when family functioning is disrupted a clinician can intervene to inform parents of a lack of communication and teach the parents developmentally appropriate ways to talk with the sibling(s) about a brother or sister's illnesses and other related family issues. The families in this study had a variety of illnesses, including obesity, cystic fibrosis, sickle cell anemia, inflammatory bowel disease and epilepsy. There were not significant differences between type of illness and family functioning.

Plumridge *et al.,* (2011) examined parental communication with siblings of children with different types of genetic conditions (*e.g.,* cystic fibrosis, neurofibromatosis, Duchene muscular dystrophy, *etc.*). Their findings revealed that for some families, communication about the fact that a sibling might be a "carrier" was poor, and there was hesitation to talk about the genetic condition in some families. Siblings with information about their brother or sister's condition were better adjusted. They cautioned that when information was not discussed, a sibling could display, "resentment or withdrawal from the affected child." (p. 379). Siblings could be very worried about their parents or brother or sister and this anxiety might intensify if the sibling feels "left out" of family communications and believes he or she does not have a role in the family. The mental health provider can assist parents in talking about the genetic condition and defining the sibling's role in the family, perhaps to be a helper and be a sibling that supports the child who has a chronic illness. Creating social family events, where "all" members have a role, can enhance family involvement, communication, and improve positive affect among family members. Stressing to parents that communication with a sibling should be ongoing, as the child and family develops, will ensure that parents are available to provide developmentally appropriate information about the child's medical condition and address different issues related to the illness. Opening communication channels makes this ongoing communication easier and more routine, which can facilitate parental abilities to engage in difficult conversations should the child's illness worsen or change.

When family functioning is impaired, referral for family counseling may be indicated. The mental health provider can observe transactions (*e.g.*, interactions) among family members and employ techniques to improve family communication and clarify roles of family members. Within family sessions, the clinician can facilitate opportunities for discussion of the illness in a safe environment, where emotions can be displayed in a supportive atmosphere. Clinicians should remain careful to "listen" to the perceptions of siblings, so that if these perceptions are inaccurate then correct medical information can be provided. Encouraging parents to have positive expectations for all children in the family can be the foundation of promoting equality and defining roles for the sibling, which can reduce sibling feelings of isolation. Graff *et al.*, (2010) assessed parent perceptions of sibling functioning when a brother or sister had sickle cell anemia. The parents reported that for the most part, sibling relationships were positive, and sibling ties were close and marked by mutual affection. However, they did note that in families where the child had a relatively high number of emergency room visits, sibling functioning could be less well-adjusted. This could be due to the severity of the child's medical condition, and thus severity of the condition and stress on the family associated with multiple medical procedures and hospitalizations remains an important variable to assess.

Another way to improve sibling functioning may be to improve support for the child at school. Alderfer and Hodges (2010) reported that siblings can feel "ignored" and they can greatly benefit from enhanced feelings of support from peers (*i.e.*, their friends at school) and their teachers. They recommended that the medical team meet with school staff or speak with them to address the special needs for support of siblings. The medical team can address sibling needs and then a school mental health professional can develop a care plan to improve support from teachers. Ideas for improving support from friends or a peer buddy could also be considered. Alderfer and Hodges were focusing on siblings with cancer, a life-threatening illness, which could have had a very significant impact on sibling functioning. In contrast, other siblings, with a brother or sister with a less severe illness, may be functioning quite well, and may not need extra planning for support at school. Sibling functioning should be evaluated on a case-by-case basis to determine if the sibling is exhibiting behavioral or emotional problems or other issues, such as increased somatic complaints. If functioning is impaired, then planning for sibling adjustment should be addressed.

COPING WITH THE DEATH OF A BROTHER OR SISTER

A special situation, involving knowledge about grief counseling, occurs when a child with a life-threatening chronic illness dies. Very young siblings may not understand what death means. Children typically have an understanding of death being permanent at approximately nine years of age. This is not absolute, however, and the clinician should carefully assess whether the sibling understands that the death of a brother or sister is permanent. Helping the child express his or her grief and being a support for the child is critical, as some parents may be grieving themselves. Therefore, they may not be as available as they usually might be to support their child. The child needs to know that coping with grief involves the resolution of many different types of feelings – such as anger, disbelief, sadness, and at times feelings of guilt over being the sibling that got to keep on living (this is known as survivor's guilt). If necessary, referral should be made for counseling for siblings having a strong grief reaction – that is very intense in nature and limits daily functioning or lasts longer than a year (Packman *et al.,* 2006).

Allowing the sibling to create a memory or way to memorialize his or her brother or sister can be a powerful way to allow the child to express his or her grief and create a meaning as he or she copes with the loss. Some of the clinical tools this author has used are having the child create a memory book – using either photographs or drawings. There can be a page for a birthday memory, your favorite thing to do with your brother or sister, the funniest day, and what I would like to remember about _____ (name of brother or sister who died). Use of memorial ceremonies, such as drumming and releasing balloons with notes or pictures can help create a new beginning where the sibling can start to conceive of the brother or sister bond as a special memory to carry forward throughout his or her life. Sometimes siblings will like to wear clothing or jewelry or keep items to remind them of their brother or sister and this can be a part of normal adjustment processes.

Packman *et al.,* (2006) wrote about the continuing bonding between a sibling and a deceased brother or sister that can last throughout a sibling's life. As such, family members should be counseled to be open to communicating about the loss at different points during the child's development. In order to help the sibling make meaning of the loss and move on with his or her life, the sibling must – "…learn the world in a way that helps one accommodate and live with the loss." (Packman *et al.,* 2006, p. 18). The brother or sister may remain a part of the sibling's identity throughout his or her life, as the sibling strives to move on and create a meaningful life that includes the sibling – in memory. However, all memories may not be positive and the bond may not be as strong or as positive for siblings who had a negative relationship (marked by conflict and sibling rivalry) and this should be considered when assisting the sibling in working through grief related to the loss of a brother or sister. Significant occasions (*e.g.,* holidays and birthdays) are times that memories can be particularly strong and even upsetting and the sibling may need extra support from family members during special occasions.

In order to understand the nature of parental support, the clinician needs to assess the parents' reaction to the loss of their child. If the parent is not open to discussing the loss or cannot cope with the loss, this stance may inadvertently impact siblings. Effects can be negative, if the sibling feels that he or she cannot express feelings of grief and other emotions related to the death of a brother or sister who had a chronic illness. The sibling may feel that he or she is "not enough" and is not able to fill his or her brother or sister's shoes. This can occur if the sibling perceived the brother or sister who died as being very talented or favored by parents or caregivers (Packman *et al.*, 2006). Another good resource for clinicians is a book by Webb (2002) entitled, "Helping Bereaved Children: A Handbook for Practitioners." In conducting an assessment of sibling functioning the mental health practitioner should make plans for assisting with grief based on: (1) characteristics of the surviving sibling, (2) the situation surrounding the loss, (3) parental and family reactions to the loss, (4) the relationship between the sibling and his or her brother or sister before the death, and (5) what is happening in the child's current context. Allowing the child to slowly and carefully work through memories and express feelings as needed, provides an atmosphere for resolution of grief issues (Packman *et al.*, 2006).

One method for making the concept of death more "understandable" for young children is to explain death in terms of lifecycles. Here's an example, "Every living thing has a time to live and a time to die. Here are examples, flowers, leaves on trees, the trees themselves, bugs, pets, and other animals. Human beings also have a time to live and a time to die. This time might be different for different living things and humans live for different periods of time. A book that may be beneficial for some young children is, "The Fall of Freddie the Leaf: A Story of Life for All Ages" by Leo Buscaglia (1982). Another book that might be helpful in improving younger children's knowledge is entitled, "Lifetimes: The Thoughtful Way to Explain Death to Children," and was written by Bryan Mellonie (1983). Both of these books review the concept of lifecycles and teach the permanency of loss in a developmentally appropriate manner.

Pediatricians often do not receive much education about grief counseling. Mental health practitioners can provide guidance in this area, as children may turn to their pediatrician for answers. Wender and the Committee on Psychosocial Aspects of Child and Family Health (2012) wrote an insightful article in *Pediatrics* that provides guidance for pediatricians and other primary care providers about how to help a sibling process the loss of a brother or sister. In this article, they review the notion that the sibling is in "mourning" and parents might not be as available as they usually might be to provide support and have open lines of communication with the sibling. In these cases, extended family can support the sibling. Similar to Packman *et al.*, (2006), Wender *et al.*, (2012) recommended that clinicians ensure that the child is able to understand that death is permanent and be ready to help the child deal with guilt regarding the loss of a brother or sister – especially if the relationship involved conflict or rivalry before the loss of the brother or sister. Wender *et al.*, (2012) advised pediatricians to determine whether the child is assuming a care-taking role, and helping them with this and reintegrating them into their role as a child in the family, if this is occurring. They recommended referral to support groups for siblings when indicated. Similarly, O'Brien *et al.*, (2009) recommended referral to support groups and provision of family support as a two-pronged intervention for caring for siblings when a child in the family is facing a chronic illness.

Forward and Garlie (2003) discussed positive adjustment of adolescents after the death of a brother or sister. First, siblings who experience loss of a brother or sister can become more sensitive and compassionate. Second, they can have more empathy for others who are in difficult situations. Third, siblings may develop life goals and strive to live life with a purpose. Fourth, they may display affection more readily. Fifth, they may be less apt to engage in risky behaviors compared to peers who have not experienced the loss of a loved one. These are positive implications that can occur if siblings resolve their grief and loss in a positive way, maintaining an ongoing positive mental connection with their brother or sister and making meaning of the relationship as they continue to move forward with their lives. Forward and Garlie focused on adolescent coping, and more research is needed with younger children to understand if they have the potential for positive character development after the loss of a brother or sister.

CASE STUDY: BOY WITH SPINA BIFIDA

Consider the functioning of the James' family where a young boy is experiencing spina bifida. There are three boys in this family and Max, the middle child, was born with spina bifida. His case is not severe; he can walk with leg braces and is doing fairly well in school. Max had very good personal hygiene and social skills and had a group of friends at school and in his neighborhood. He did have some emotional outbursts at home, typically related to not being able to play basketball or soccer with his older brother and other boys in the neighborhood. Max's behavior at school was considered "perfect" he was a "model citizen" and always followed directions and completed his work on time. This was not the case at home. Max sometimes "tested" his mother and did not follow her instructions. He did better with his father, listening to his directives and sharing his feelings, which resulted in tension in Max's relationship with his mother, who was his primary caretaker.

Max's mother called for counseling to improve Max's behavior at home and to learn about strategies for coping with his angry outbursts. His mother felt that she was "inadequate" in terms of disciplining Max, and that their interactions could result in yelling and an exchange of angry words. Max often would not go to his room to "take a time out" so that he could manage his emotions. This resulted in angry exchanges that disrupted positive family functioning and typically ended in a call to Max's father who would discipline Max, by sending him to his room, when he came home. This was starting to place strain on Max and his father's relationship and his younger brother was feeling that "Max gets all the attention" because he always was acting "bad" at home.

The counselor began with recording information about Max and his brothers' developmental histories which were within normal limits and without significant developmental or medical incidents or problems. Relations among parents were good; they had open communication and supported each other in decisions about child-rearing. They did tend to withhold information from siblings about Max's condition so as not to "burden them" with knowledge that would lead to worry and stress. The youngest sibling, Luke, was developing normally. However; recently, he had begun mimicking Max's outbursts in interactions with his mother, especially when he wanted to go outside to play with friends and his mother asked him to finish his school work before playing.

The counselor began with a parenting session with mother and father to address Max and Luke's outbursts. They talked about use of natural and logical consequences, such as not being able to go outside and play until homework was completed and interactions with their mother were positive in nature. This intervention worked for Max, but Luke continued to have difficulty with following his mother's instructions. He seemed to be angry with Max and reported that "Max gets all the attention." Luke was still doing well at school, and like his brother Max he was a model citizen – exhibiting good behavior and getting good grades at school. Luke also had a group of friends at school and in the neighborhood. He was involved in soccer, which he particularly enjoyed, as an extracurricular activity. In the spring he was looking forward to joining a local baseball team, which his father would coach. Thus, his problem was circumscribed, limited to poor interactions with his mother and negative mood at home. Luke was eating and sleeping well and getting along well with his father and both of his brothers. He did, however, occasionally express to them that he felt "left out" because Max always had medical visits with their mother and got lots of attention from their mother and father.

After learning about Luke's concerns, the counselor suggested that his mother and father schedule a special time with Luke to explain Max's condition to him and let him know that the condition necessitated many medical visits. They discussed finding a role for Luke, in terms of improving his involvement in family activities. The role that they selected was "planner" in that Luke would take a lead role in planning family activities on the weekends. Luke would develop ideas for family activities based on interviewing family members and writing down ideas on a white board posted in the kitchen.

In terms of discipline, the counselor introduced the idea of "time outs" taken by the mother (to withdraw attention from Luke). These time outs would involve mother walking away and withdrawing her attention from Luke if he became angry and had an outburst. She would return and pay attention to Luke when his behavior had become appropriate. Of course, Luke's safety would be assured and these "Mommy time outs" would occur only in those situations where Luke was safe. Thus, the loss of attention from his mother was considered a mild punishment for inappropriate behaviors that the counselor suspected were driven, in part, in an effort to gain more of his mother's attention.

The counselor and parents met to determine the success of their ideas after two weeks. Luke had benefitted from learning about his brother's medical condition. He had expressed sympathy and shown more understanding of the need for medical visits. Luke asked to come along and he had joined Max and his mother on two medical visits. On one of these visits, Luke had an opportunity to talk with Max's doctor. Luke seemed more at ease with the attention Max was receiving after he learned more information about Max's medical condition.

The maternal time outs did not initially meet with success, but over the long-term they started to work, and after three weeks, Luke's mother called the counselor and stated that Luke had made great improvements in getting angry with her when she gave him directions. He no longer yelled and became angry when asked to do his homework or a chore. He talked about not liking, "Mom going away." His mother and Luke began spending special time together (10 minutes every evening) where his mother played whatever Luke selected or talked with him about his interests. Luke's behavior toward his mother rapidly improved in the upcoming weeks, and his angry outbursts extinguished or stopped. Luke looked forward to special time, which would occur even if he did not behave well. His improved communication and relationship with his mother resulted in improved mood for both Luke and his mother and smoother family functioning, as his father did not have to assume the role of disciplinarian after he had returned home from a long day of work. Luke's mother's attitude improved and she became more confident in her parenting skills and felt better about her role as a parent.

CONCLUSION

This chapter focused on a review of sibling functioning when a brother or sister has a chronic illness. Information on how siblings can feel was reviewed as well as ideas for improving family communication and sibling functioning. In general, siblings are "at risk" for adjustment problems when a brother or sister has a chronic illness (Vermaes *et al.*, 2012). Siblings can feel isolated and "left out" in terms of having a key role in the family (Alderfer & Hodges, 2010; Graff *et al.*, 2010). Identifying ideas for improving sibling knowledge of the brother or sister's medical condition is one intervention for improving sibling understanding and functioning within the family. Defining a role for a sibling within the family unit can help the sibling adjust to the stress of having a brother or sister with a chronic illness. Opening family communication is a developmental goal that needs to continue as the family, sibling, and child with the illness grow and change (Besier *et al.*, 2010; Herzer *et al.*, 2010; Plumridge *et al.*, 2011). Keeping communication open can provide an avenue to improve understanding of the waxing and waning nature of chronic illness and a channel for discussing negative events that might impact the family.

There are examples of interventions to improve sibling functioning (*e.g.*, Lobato & Kao, 2002). Involving both the parent and sibling in the intervention – and ensuring that support groups are provided – can ensure the success of an intervention in improving sibling and family functioning. On the other hand, there is a dearth of research on interventions to enhance sibling functioning and further research addressing the long-term effects of interventions on sibling functioning will advance knowledge in the field. Supporting parents can also improve sibling functioning, as interactions and transactions in the family are reciprocal. Improving parent functioning, knowledge, and abilities to communicate with children can have a positive impact on the sibling and entire family (Lemarche & Newton, 2012; Plumridge *et al.*, 2011). Finally, ensuring that the sibling has support at school, in cases where parent stress is high, can ensure support for a distressed sibling (Alderfer & Hodges, 2010).

Death of a brother or sister with a life-threatening condition is a tremendous stress on the family unit. Counseling can be indicated in this situation. In order to help a child understand the concept of death, discussion of lifecycles can be important. Providing support for parents and understanding how to provide grief counseling is an important skill for the mental health provider (Webb, 2002; Wender *et al.*, 2012). Siblings can adjust positively, showing increased compassion for others after a family loss (Forward & Garlie, 2003). Part of successful adaptation to loss is finding a way to understand the "reason" for the loss and finding ways to go on with life and build new life meaning that considers the life and contribution of a brother or sister who has died because of a chronic illness. Grief reactions typically last a year, and the counselor needs to be present for the family, in order to be available if a severe grief reaction occurs and ongoing support of the sibling and family is needed.

ACKNOWLEDGEMENTS

None declared.

CONFLICT OF INTEREST

The author confirms that this chapter contents have no conflict of interest.

REFERENCES

Alderfer, M. A., & Hodges, J. A. (2010). Supporting siblings of children with cancer: A need for family-school partnerships. *School Mental Health, 2*(2), 72-81.

Alderfer, M. A., Labay, L. E., & Kazak, A. E. (2003). Brief report: Does posttraumatic stress apply to siblings of childhood cancer survivors? *Journal of Pediatric Psychology, 28*, 281-286.

Besier, T., Hölling, H., Schlack, R., West, C., & Goldback, L. (2010). Impact of a family-oriented rehabilitation programme on behavioral and emotional problems in healthy siblings of chronically ill children. *Child: Care, Health and Development, 36*(5), 686-695.

Buscaglia, L. F. (1982). *The Fall of Freddie the Leaf: A Story of Life for All Ages.* Thorofare, N. J.: SLACK.

Forward, D. R., & Garlie, N. (2003). Search for new meaning: Adolescent bereavement after the sudden death of a sibling. *Canadian Journal of School Psychology, 18*(1-2), 23-53.

Gilmore, L., Waugh, M., Haynes, A., Hearne, C., Mercer, C., & Wilson, K. (2012). Supporting siblings of children with a rare chromosome disorder. *Unique*, pp. 1-8, http://eprints.qut.edu/au/52927.

Gold, J. I., Treadwell, M., Weissman, L., & Vichinsky, E. (2011). The mediating effects of family functioning on psychosocial outcomes in healthy siblings of children with sickle cell disease. *Pediatric Blood Cancer, 57*, 1055-1061.

Graff, J. C., Hankins, J. S., Hardy, B. T., Hull, H. R., Roberts, R. J., & Neely-Barns, S. L. (2010). Exploring parent-sibling communication in families of children with sickle cell disease. *Issues in Comprehensive Pediatric Nursing, 33*(2), 101-123.

Hames, A., & Appleton, R. (2009). Living with a brother or sister with epilepsy: Siblings' experiences. *Seizure: European Journal of Epilepsy, 18*(10), 699-701. DOI: 10.1016/j.seizure.2009.10.002.

Herzer, M., Godiwala, N., Hommel, K. A., Driscoll, K., Mitchell, M., Crosby, L., Piazza-Wagoner, C., Zeller, M. H., & Modi, A. C. (2010). Family functioning in the context of pediatric chronic conditions. *Journal of Developmental and Behavioral Pediatrics, 31*(1), 26-34.

Lemarche, K., & Newton, K. (2012). Take the challenge: Strategies to improve support for parents of chronically ill children. *Home Healthcare Nurse, 30*(5), E1-E8. http://www.nursingcenter.com/lnc/Static-Pages/Take-the-Challenge-Strategies-to-Improve-Support-f.

Lobato, D. J., & Kao, B. T. (2002). Integrated sibling and parent group intervention to improve sibling knowledge and adjustment to chronic illness and disability. *Journal of Pediatric Psychology, 27*(8), 711-716.

Mellonie, B. (1983). *Lifetimes: The thoughtful way to explain death to children.* New York: Bentham Publishers.

Menke, E. M. (1987). The impact of a child's chronic illness on school-aged siblings. *Children's Health Care, 15*(3), 132-140.

Neilson, K. M., Mandleco, B., Roper, S. O., Cox, A., Dyches, T., & Marshall, E. S. (2012). Parental perceptions of sibling relationships in families rearing a child with a chronic condition. *Journal of Pediatric Nursing, 27*, 34-43.

Plumridge, G., Metcalfe, A., Coad, J., & Gill, P. (2011). Parents' communication with siblings of children affected by an inherited condition. *Journal of Genetic Counseling, 20*(4), 374-383.

O'Brien, I., Duffy, A., & Nicholl, H. (2009). Impact of childhood chronic illnesses on siblings: A literature review. *British Journal of Nursing, 18*(22), 1358-1365.

O'Haver, J., Moore, I. M., Insel, K. C., Reed, P. G., Melnyk, B. M., & Lavoie, M. (2010). Parental perceptions of risk and protective factors associated with the adaptation of siblings of children with cystic fibrosis. *Pediatric Nursing, 36*(3), 284-291.

Packman, W., Horsley, H., Davies, B., & Kramer, R. (2006). Sibling bereavement and continuing bonds. *Death Studies, 30*, 817-841.

Redshaw, S., & Wilson, V. (2012). Sibling involvement in childhood chronic heart disease through a bead program. *Journal of Child Health Care, 16*(1), 53-61.

Vermaes, I. P. R., van Susante, A. M., & van Bakel, H. J. A. (2012). *Journal of Pediatric Psychology, 37*(2), 166-184.

Waite-Jones, J. M., & Madill, A., (2008). Amplified ambivalence: Having a sibling with juvenile idiopathic arthritis. *Psychology and Health, 23*(4), 477-492.

Webb, N. B. (2002). *Helping bereaved children: A handbook for practitioners.* New York: Guilford Press.

Wender, E., & the Committee on Psychosocial Aspects of Child and Family Health (2012). Supporting the family after the death of a child. *Pediatrics, 130*, 1164-1169.

Williams, P. D., Ridder, E. L., Setter, R. K., Liebergen, A., Curry, H., Piamjariyakul, U., & Williams, A. R. (2009). Pediatric chronic illness (cancer, cystic fibrosis) effects on well siblings: Parents' voices. *Issues in Comprehensive Pediatric Nursing, 32*, 94-113.

CHAPTER 9

Transition to Adult Medical Care

Laura A. Nabors[*]

Health Education Program, School of Human Services, University of Cincinnati, 468 Dyer Hall, Mail Location 0068, Cincinnati, Ohio, OH 45221-0068, USA

Abstract: The transition to adult health care providers and specialists can be very stressful for young adults who have essentially "grown up" with their pediatric health care team. Respecting the close bonds that can form between pediatric providers and their young patients and families is critical. Involving the pediatric team in the transition planning and process is important and can facilitate both child success and the education of the adult care providers. Allowing youth to learn about adult care and perhaps even having a practice visit with an adult provider can facilitate their transition process. Others have suggested that having transition clinics may be a method for providing health care for this special age group. Having a portable medical summary with contact information for reaching the pediatric care team is recommended. Helping the young adult understand the "ins and outs" of his or her insurance plan and assisting him or her as he or she assumes responsibility for self-management are other actions to assist the young adult. When adult providers adopt a family-centered as well as a patient-centered model of care they can address concerns of the family unit. This orientation may be helpful as the family and young adult are a long-standing team and may be coping with the transition to adult health care as a unit.

Keywords: Family-centered approach, medical summary, self-management; transition, understanding insurance, young adulthood.

INTRODUCTION

A key developmental transition for the child who has a chronic illness is the move to adult medical care. Transitioning to adult health care is an important area of study for all young adults, especially for individuals with special health care needs (U.S. Department of Health and Human Services, 2000). McDonagh (2005) stated that that transition to adult care represents a "…process that attends to the

---

*Address correspondence to Laura A. Nabors: Health Education Program, School of Human Services, University of Cincinnati, 468 Dyer Hall, Mail Location 0068, Cincinnati, Ohio, OH 45221-0068, USA; Tel: 513-556-5537; Fax: 513-556-3898; E-mail: naborsla@ucmail.uc.edu

medical, psychological, and educational/vocational needs of adolescents as they move from child to adult centered care" (p. 364). The transition from pediatric to adult care for those with chronic illnesses and special health care needs can be difficult (Binks *et al.*, 2007; Lotstein *et al.*, 2005; National Center for Youth with Disabilities, 1995). Finding an adult physician or medical team and helping the young adult and family members adjust to the differences in health care may be a change that a mental health provider can assist with.

Children with chronic illnesses may elect to remain with their pediatric medical care team, because they have formed close relationships with this team and believe that they have the specialized knowledge of best practices in terms of how to care for their medical issues. A well-timed transition to adult health care is recommended between the ages of eighteen to twenty-one years and the planning process begins in adolescence (Cooley *et al.*, 2011; Reiss *et al.*, 2005). The mental health provider can play a key role in helping the child and his or her parents "think through" the pros and cons of the decision to remain with the current medical team or transition to working with an adult team.

The adolescent and his or her family may need guidance and support in transitioning from high school to college. Connecting with staff and explaining the medical condition in higher education settings can be stressful. Typically, the office for students with special needs or disabilities can assist the young adult with developing a plan to provide things like, extra time on tests and opportunities to complete work missed due to medical illness. Other services could include having note-takers, taking tests in individual settings, and plans for making up school work due to hospitalizations resulting in extended absences. The transition process should begin with an assessment of patient and family readiness, which also considers the youth's educational and vocational needs, abilities for independent living and self-advocacy, and capacity to adhere to his or her medical regimen (Cooley *et al.*, 2011).

Adolescents with medical conditions may experience difficulty transitioning to college and feel that their quality of life, health, or health care may suffer during this transition period. For example, Boyle *et al.*, (2001) reported that adolescents with cystic fibrosis were concerned that their health care quality would suffer when they transitioned to college and needed to find a new, adult health care team. Reiss and Gibson (2002) stated that youth with chronic illnesses and their parents often feel that the children's health suffered in their adult years, because adult physicians and medical teams did not deliver the same quality of care that pediatric health care teams provided. Results are not clear-cut, however. Others have shown that transition to an adult health care provider has health benefits for college students who have chronic medical conditions (Lotstein *et al.*, 2005). McDonagh (2005) reviewed literature on transitions for young adults with chronic illnesses and reported that most young adults would prefer to meet their new adult care team prior to an initial appointment and prior to accepting them as their adult health care providers.

Stewart (2009) reviewed ideas for a successful transition to adult care for young adults with disabilities. She recommended collaboration between providers to ensure that the transition occurs and to coordinate service delivery. Stewart mentioned that in addition to education of the young adults, it is critical to educate physicians. Physicians who primarily work in the field of pediatrics need to understand key transition issues and health risks for young adults. Physicians need to understand that their support and their discussion of the transition are critical to the success of the transition process for many youth (Binks *et al.*, 2007; Stewart, 2009). Similarly, young adults need to be able to describe their chronic illness to their new team -- in their own words (McDonagh, 2005). A role for the mental health provider may be to practice with the youth, using role play exercises, explaining his or her illness to others. Some other key areas to review with the adolescent include being able to describe the illness, being comfortable letting others know about the illness, and overcoming hesitancy to tell teachers, supervisors, new friends and significant others about the illness.

STUDIES ASSESSING THE TRANSITION TO ADULT CARE

A study conducted by Wodka and Barakat (2007) examined the role of family support and coping in the adjustment of adolescents with a chronic illness and their transition to college. The group of students they studied reported more anxiety and tendencies toward depression compared to the healthy students. This study showed that transition is more challenging for those with other life stressors such as a chronic illness. Social support has been shown to minimize or buffer the effects of stress in adolescence. Specifically, research has found that students who perceive they have an adequate amount of social support report their quality of life, health, and their health care as better than those who perceive a relatively low amount of social support. For many students the transition to college presents a very important developmental challenge in taking care of their health and having a good quality of life. Many adolescents handle this transition to college successfully; however, there is evidence that a subset of the population has difficulty. A significant minority of students suffering from a chronic illness may have a harder time during the transition than other healthy students who are transitioning to young adulthood (Wodka & Barakat, 2007).

Tuchman and Schwartz (2013) compared transition to adulthood for patients with cystic fibrosis who remained with their pediatric health care team to those who transferred to adult health care teams. Their findings did not indicate significant differences on health care variables, showing positive health outcomes for both groups. Tuchman and Schwartz commented that their findings contrasted with those of other studies which could show negative outcomes when youth with cystic fibrosis transitioned to adult services.

In an earlier paper, Tuchman *et al.*, (2010) outlined ideas for ensuring a transition that would yield positive health outcomes for young adults with cystic fibrosis. They discussed the importance of having a coordinator, who managed the transition process, to help the youth and his or her family. They suggested that, in order to combat the lack of adult care providers, more physicians may need to be recruited and trained to provide transition services for young adults with cystic fibrosis. Moreover, the team's coordinator may need to advise and help the youth and his or her family understand new insurance plans and help the young adult read the "fine print" detailing service provision.

Similar to other experts (*e.g.*, Cooley *et al.*, 2011), Tuchman *et al.*, (2010) recommended a continual assessment process to determine whether the adolescent to adult health care transition yielded patient satisfaction as well as positive health outcomes. One problem unique to those with cystic fibrosis is concerns related to infection control. Keeping patients isolated, so that the spread of infection is controlled could contribute to feelings of isolation for young adults. Developing online support groups and educational webcasts may be a way to educate and provide support to young adults with cystic fibrosis. Tuchman *et al.*, (2010) also pointed out that establishing adult centers is important, as more youth with cystic fibrosis are living longer, and therefore as adults they are faced with more medical complications and deteriorating health, which can increase the burden of care at a time when they are beginning to take over their disease management.

Reiss *et al.*, (2005) conducted 34 focus groups with youth and young adults with chronic illnesses and disabilities, family members, and members of the medical team. These groups were conducted in nine different cities in the Southern and Midwestern regions of the United States. The different "interest groups" were in separate focus groups, which allowed for free expression of the pros and cons about the transition to adult medical care. The focus group format allowed the researchers to explore opinions and perceptions of the nature of the relationship between the pediatric health care team, children, and families. These relationships were described as close bonds and the transition process should be handled with care to recognize these close ties and the need to slowly transition to adult services. One problem was that some perceived pediatric services as ending abruptly without offering opportunities to celebrate the relationship and offer opportunities for closure.

Results from the focus groups suggested that adult teams could be perceived as less available for support and questions (Reiss *et al.*, 2005). It may be that conversations between the pediatric and adult care team can assist the adult providers in learning about the child's disease and its management, as well as providing them with a glimpse of the importance of a "family-centered" care model for the successful treatment of youth with chronic illnesses. Reiss *et al.*, (2005) highlighted the process of transition as having three major stages. The first, envisioning the transition, begins early and the age at which discussion of the transition begins can differ given the developmental stage of the youth and his or her family. The second stage is determining when the adolescent is ready to assume more self-care and self-management of his or her illness. The third stage is the age of transition, when the young person is developmentally ready to assume a more independent role in disease management. Considering where the youth and family are positioned, in terms of the aforementioned stages, provides a process-oriented guide for review of information and developing transition planning based on adolescent or young adult and family readiness to make changes.

KEY TOPICS FOR DISCUSSION WITH YOUNG ADULTS AND THEIR PARENTS

Lotstein *et al.*, (2009) assessed planning for the transition to adult health care using data from the 2005-2006 National Survey of Children with Special Healthcare Needs. They discovered that children with special health care needs can experience difficulty finding health care and feeling comfortable with their medical providers as they "age out" of their children's health services. Topics that need to be addressed include: (1) the shift to an adult provider, (2) what the youth's future health care needs will be, (3) insurance opportunities available in adulthood (after the youth transitions from parent or caregiver insurance), and (4) improving youth involvement in self-management of illness and assuming responsibility for self-care. Discussions about vocational or college planning should begin as the student finishes middle school or when the youth is about thirteen years of age.

Parents might welcome discussions, but at times pediatric providers may be hesitant to discuss future options, because they are unsure of what these will be. Lotstein *et al.*, (2009) may have underestimated the amount of conversations occurring between pediatricians and young adults about transitions. However, they used parent self-report data and pediatricians could be having private conversations with youth about their transitions to adult health providers. Those children who were uninsured, from low-income families, and who had more severe health problems or illnesses were less likely to be informed and be engaged in transition conversations, indicating that this is an area for future research and intervention (Lotstein *et al.*, 2009).

Addressing adolescent self-advocacy, by teaching the adolescent to be aware of and support his or her rights and needs can be a key task, given that parents have served in that role for a long period of time. Planning for a transition to independent living is critical, and can be challenging if a parent or parents are used to caring for their child's needs (Cooley *et al.*, 2011; McDonagh, 2005). Along with independence and needs for self-advocacy come major changes in the burden of care. It is advantageous for the pediatric team to plan for co-management or shared disease management during adolescence in order to make the transition to self-management in young adulthood smoother. Utilizing a "guided" decision-making process where parents and the child co-manage illness decisions and planning may be a good way to begin the transition of responsibility for disease management to the young adult. The guided decision-making should continue until the adolescent is "ready" to assume more responsibility. Furthermore, the mental health practitioner can assess parent functioning, as many parents face uncertainty and a sense of loss as their child transitions to self-management of his or her illness and life in young adulthood.

Continued assessment of adolescent and parent readiness and ability to transition to an adult care model is a component of the movement from adolescent to adult health care (Cooley *et al.*, 2011). Providing educational materials for the adolescent and his or her family can be beneficial. Fact sheets, detailing steps for a smooth transition process can be valuable instructional tools for the youth and his or her parents (McManus *et al.*, 2008). Addressing problems related to interagency coordination and coordination of adult services, before the young adult transitions to new providers may ease the transition process (McDonagh, 2005).

Using a measure to assess youth readiness may be an ideal method for assessing readiness and gathering information that will serve as conversation topics with young adults and their family members. Sawicki *et al.*, (2011) developed the *Transition Readiness Assessment Questionnaire* (*TRAQ*), and this instrument has good psychometric properties on initial review. This measure examines youth and young adults' perceptions of key issues related to successful transition to adult health care. Table **1** summarizes some of the key areas addressed by the *TRAQ*.

Future research should address the predictive validity of questionnaires, such as the *TRAQ*, in predicting young adults' adjustment to adult health care and adult living. These types of measures can also be used to assess the success of the transition process in longitudinal studies and in research assessing educational and supportive interventions to improve the transition to adult health care.

Table 1:   Assessing Readiness for the Transition to Adult Care

Area	Items to Assess
Adherence	Diet, Exercise, Medication – is independent management possible? What degree of support is needed? Can the patient reorder medication and afford self-care independently?
Access	Does the patient have transportation – can he or she get to the doctors' offices? Can the patient make their own appointments and show for appointments? Is the patient able to talk to doctors on his or her own?
Independent Living	Cooking, housekeeping, vocational and education needs met?
Advocacy	Can the patient tell others about healthcare needs?
Support	Areas: Financial, Insurance, Family, Friends, and Community.

OVERCOMING BARRIERS TO THE TRANSITION TO ADULT SERVICES

Barriers to the transition process should be identified and then reviewed with the youth, parent, and pediatric providers. The mental health clinician should be aware of these barriers and be part of a planning process that finds ways to overcome barriers and develop an optimal health transition for the young adult. McManus *et al.*, (2008) identified several barriers toward moving to adult health care for adolescents with special health care needs. For instance, a shortage of adult providers and fragmentation of services can be an impediment to a transition from the pediatric team, where a host of specialty services are available for "one-stop" shopping at the children's hospital. Navigating the adult insurance system can be overwhelming for some young adults with chronic illnesses.

Close ties and bonds between the pediatric team and the child need to be considered as well. Over time the team can develop close ties with the child and family and both sides can feel a sense of loss when the child needs to transition to adult providers. Moreover, parents can experience a loss of purpose and a loss of self as they are no longer the primary caregiver for their child (Cooley *et al.*, 2011). Several financial barriers can impede the transition process. Pediatric and adult care teams can experience a loss of funding, due to lack of reimbursement for transition planning and services (McManus *et al.*, 2008). Developing a portable health summary record for the young adult to transfer to multiple health care providers can be a support for providing medical information and recommendations for new providers (Cooley *et al.*, 2011). Establishing a transition clinic or separate clinic for young adults to learn about their care in adulthood may be advantageous and ensure feelings of "fit" and "match" with new adult roles (Crowley *et al.*, 2011).

Crowley *et al.*, (2011) found that interventions that were successful typically focused on education of the youth, careful staffing of the transition team or providing a transition medical home, and follow-up of the young adult's progress during the transition process. Young adults may feel uncomfortable in adult clinics and feel "out of place" (Crowley *et al.*, 2011). Adult providers see patients in a wide age range, and some youth may be less comfortable when introduced to adult care in clinics with patients of all ages, some of whom may be older and as a consequence are coping with significant negative health outcomes. Establishing a transition clinic, only for young adults, can help them begin to feel a sense of place with their new medical team (Binks *et al.*, 2007). Meetings between a transition coordinator, perhaps a member of the pediatric medical team, and the adult health care team can also eliminate emotional barriers to developing a bond with adult providers. It may help to develop a single contact person to overcome young adults' resistance to transition because they are overwhelmed with the "separated" or individualized service providers for different types of specialty care for adults. The mental health provider could serve as the point of contact for questions about transition and a representative that maintains contact with both the pediatric and adult team as an adult health care plan is established. Gradual connection to adult providers, so that the young adult can become comfortable and establish a sense of a new medical home could be beneficial (Crowley *et al.*, 2011).

Dowshen and D'Angelo (2011) wrote about transition planning for young adults with HIV/AIDS. They noted that transition to adult services and continued care in adulthood is needed due to the tremendous medical advances ensuring longevity for youth with HIV/AIDS. Assessment needs for young adults with HIV/AIDS are unique. In addition to assessing satisfaction and health outcomes, it is necessary to assess for change in cognitive functioning and possible problems with emotional and behavioral functioning, chiefly problems with anxiety and depression. Dowshen and D'Angelo recommended coaching and support to assist the young adult as he or she transitions to adult health care providers. Establishing psychosocial support, either through a team or mental health provider, can be a key component of good care, and the mental health provider can ensure a smooth transition process as well as assist the young adult with developing adherence plans for taking medication and attending appointments. Specialists in adult care also should be prepared to address sexual and reproductive health education and counseling.

Reid *et al.*, (2004) provided information about the transition to adult health care for three hundred and sixty young adults between the ages of nineteen to twenty-one years who had congenital heart defects. They reported that one hundred and seventy of the youth had transferred to adult heart clinics. Variables related to the likelihood of transitioning were having more serious procedures related to heart problems, having talked with the pediatrician or pediatric team about transitioning, and patient perception that follow-up care in adulthood should be in an adult clinic where providers specialize in heart defects. Youth with congenital heart problems need specialty follow-up care (every year to two years) in case previous problems recur and because they are at risk for early mortality. Because of the serious long-term risks, Reid *et al.*, (2004) stressed the importance of early communication between doctors, children, and parents about the need for specialty care and follow-up in the young adult years and beyond.

QUALITY OF CARE AND COLLABORATION DRIVING THE TRANSITION PROCESS

White *et al.*, (2012) developed a review paper that offers a great model for approaching the transition process from a quality improvement approach. They mentioned that only 40% of youth with chronic conditions are receiving the transition support that they need, making quality improvement efforts in the transition to adult health services a key area for improvement of patient care. They recommended that pediatric teams develop a portable medical summary of the youth's illness and its management. Youth should experience the adult medical system for a practice session around 18 years of age. They may benefit from support from their pediatric team as they learn to navigate the adult health care system. The young adult should be educated about how to create a more family-friendly model of care, if he or she wants this model, through providing permission to involve family members consistent with HIPPA privacy rules. Pediatric and adult providers should review guidelines provided by the National Healthcare Transition Center. Among the guidelines provided by this center are: the importance of planning for and practicing transition, developing a registry of youth who will need extra support with transition, and providing written care plans to support the transition processes for these patients and their families. They recommended collaboration be at the center of the relationship between the adult and pediatric care teams and that both adopt a quality improvement model to ensure the highest standards of medical care for the young adult.

CASE STUDY: GIRL WITH TYPE I DIABETES

Molly is a 15-year-old girl with Type I Diabetes. She currently is seen monthly, by a mental health provider, for support in adhering to her medical regimen. At times, Molly has had some difficulty with counting carbohydrates and using her pump, especially when she feels pressure to appear "normal," when coping with peer pressure. Molly's parents have kept a tight watch on her insulin administration through interrogating her pump. They assist her with counting carbohydrates and remembering to "test" her blood sugar regularly. Sometimes Molly believes this oversight is "nagging" and occasional visits to her therapist involve family sessions to address adolescent-parent tensions.

At a recent visit, Molly's therapist had an opportunity to discuss her transition to adult care. Molly had mentioned that she was "feeling frustrated" with the oversight and assistance offered by her mother. At the same time, she did admit that her blood sugar levels had been "all over the place" and she did not always test her blood glucose levels on a regular basis, as she was "supposed to do." Molly's counselor talked about her mother's perspective – which included worry that Molly would not take care of her diabetes, and then in the long run would suffer from negative health effects of not caring for her diabetes. Molly reported she had not really considered her mother's point of view.

After she admitted this, Molly and her counselor engaged in a "practice" role play, where Molly was the doctor and the therapist played the role of Molly. Prior to the beginning of the role play, the counselor provided coaching to Molly – to review key ideas for discussion of the transition to adult care. This "practice" was a non-threatening way to teach Molly about important transition issues --- such as engaging in more self-management and improving her adherence to her medical regimen (*i.e.*, glucose testing, counting carbohydrates and adjusting her insulin levels). Molly admitted she was apt to rely on her mother for taking care of her diabetes. The counselor and Molly talked about Molly needing to begin to assume more of a central role in caring for her diabetes.

Molly reluctantly agreed that learning about self-care might be beneficial – "since soon I will be in college and will not be residing in the same state as my parents." Molly and her counselor began compiling a list of diabetes management tasks and what time of day and how these procedures worked. They also identified who was in charge of "making sure" Molly counted her carbs, gave herself the right bolus (for her pump), and tested her blood glucose regularly. When Molly looked at their notes she exclaimed, "Wow, Mom is doing everything and she does too much!" Molly's mother attended the next session. After talking with the counselor and beginning to define her role as the caretaker, Molly's mother noticed that "I am doing too much and it's not helping Molly learn what she can do to take care of her diabetes." Together they developed a calendar where they divided diabetes management activities with Molly taking a greater role after a month of watching and learning from her mother. Molly hesitantly agreed to the shared management approach. She and her mother met weekly with the counselor. With encouragement from her therapist and mother, Molly was eventually able to assume many self-management tasks. Molly even began driving herself to appointments and communicated on her own with the medical team, relaying information to her mother.

Toward the end of her junior year in high school, the medical team began searching for an adult provider for Molly to visit. She met with this provider with a nurse from her pediatric medical team and learned about the steps and processes in adult medical care. Molly also had a portable summary report of her health care with the numbers of two contacts from the pediatric team who could familiarize her adult team with her previous treatment. Times were arranged for team members from the old and new teams to talk about Molly's past and current medical care. With help from her pediatric medical team and her counselor she identified doctors who could help her in her senior year of college. Molly met her doctor and specialists at a nearby university hospital. She felt like she had a medical home and had her appointments scheduled prior to leaving for college, which helped to ensure a smoother transition to her new medical home.

Molly processed feelings of sadness, related to leaving her pediatric team, who had played such a large role in helping her understand and manage her diabetes. Being able to talk about the transition and concern over the loss of the close ties allowed Molly to voice her concerns. Selecting a doctor, visiting before college began, and then scheduling appointments in advance of college starting was helpful for Molly. She understood that she could reschedule appointments, if a scheduled class or lab meeting coincided with an appointment, and she had met the medical assistant she could call to reschedule appointments. Molly knew the process for contacting her new doctor should she experience a medical problem or if she had any questions. This preparation further bolstered her confidence.

CONCLUSION

The negative effects of health conditions are reduced when individuals report satisfaction with their quality of life and positive perceptions of their health quality (Covic *et al*., 2004; Stam *et al*., 2006). Young adults' perceptions of their health quality also are related to their achievement of developmental milestones in adulthood, such as college graduation (Zullig *et al*., 2005; Stam *et al*., 2006). Asprey and Nash (2006) reported that young adults with chronic illness may report lower quality of life in the college years. This may be influenced by a host of factors, and one of the factors that may be related to lower perceptions of quality of life may be a lack of access to a specialized medical team to provide illness-specific care (Asprey & Nash, 2006; Boyle *et al*., 2001). Transition planning, as the adolescent nears the end of high school, should include plans for transition to adult health care teams with illness-specific knowledge (Lotstein *et al*., 2005). Information about factors related to having a positive adjustment to the transition to an adult health care provider and medical home for youth with serious health conditions will contribute to the literature and is an area for future research. Stewart (2009) mentioned that transition services need to be evaluated and their impact assessed over time, in longitudinal studies.

ACKNOWLEDGEMENTS

None declared.

CONFLICT OF INTEREST

The author confirms that this chapter contents have no conflict of interest.

REFERENCES

Asprey, A., & Nash, T. (2006). The importance of awareness and communication for the inclusion of young people with life-limiting and life-threatening conditions in mainstream schools and colleges. *British Journal of Special Education, 33*, 10-18.

Binks, J. A., Barden, W. S., Burke, T. A., & Young, N. L. (2007). What do we really know about the transition to adult-centered health care? A focus on cerebral palsy and spina bifida. *Archives of Physical Medicine and Rehabilitation, 88*(8), 1064-1073.

Boyle, M. P., Farukhi, Z., & Nosky, M. L. (2001). Strategies for improving transition to adult cystic fibrosis care, based on patient and parent views. *Pediatric Pulmonology, 32*, 428-436.

Cooley, C. W., Sagerman, P. J., and the American Academy of Pediatrics, American Academy of Family Physicians, and American College of Physicians, and the Transitions Clinical Report Authoring Group (2011). Supporting the health care transition from adolescence to adulthood in the medical home. *Pediatrics, 128*, 182-200. DOI: 10.1542/peds.2011-0969.

Covic, A., Seica, A., Gusbeth-Tatomir, P., Gavrilovici, O., & Goldsmith, D. J. A. (2004). Illness representations and quality of life scores in haemodialysis patients. *Nephrology, Dialysis, Transplantation, 19*, 2078-2083.

Crowley, R., Wolfe, I., Lock, K., & McKee, M. (2011). Improving the transition between paediatric and adult healthcare: A systematic review. *Archives of Disease in Childhood, 96*(6), 548-553.

Dowshen, N., & D'Angelo, L. (2011). Health care transition for youth living with HIV/AIDS. *Pediatrics, 128*(4), 762-771.

Lotstein, D. S., Ghandour, R., Cash, A., McGuire, E., Strickland, B., & Newacheck, P. (2009). Planning for health care transitions: Results from the 2005-2006 National Survey of Children with Special Healthcare Needs. *Pediatrics, 123*, e145-e152. DOI: 10.1542/peds.2008-1298.

Lotstein, D. S., McPherson, M., Strickland, B., & Newacheck, P. W. (2005). Transition planning for youth with special healthcare needs: Results from the national survey of children with special healthcare needs. *Pediatrics, 115*, 1562-1568.

McDonagh, J. E. (2005). Growing up and moving on: transition from pediatric to adult care. *Pediatric Transplantation, 9*(3), 364-372.

McManus, M., Fox, H., O'Connor, K., Chapman, T., & Mackinnon, J. (2008). *Pediatric perspectives and practice on transitioning adolescents with special needs to adult health care. Fact Sheet-No. 6, October, 2008.* National Alliance to Advance Adolescent Health: Washington, D.C.

National Center for Youth with Disabilities (1995). *Transition from child to adult health care services: A national survey.* The National Center for Youth with Disabilities, University of Minnesota, Box 721, 420 Delaware St. SE, Minneapolis, MN 55455.

Reid, G. J., Irvine, M. J., McCrindle, B. W., Sananes, R., Ritvo, P. G., Siu, S. C., & Webb, G. D. (2004). Prevalence and correlates of successful transfer from pediatric to adult health care among a cohort of young adults with complex congenital heart defects. *Pediatrics, 113*(3), e197-e205.

Reiss, J., & Gibson, R. (2002). Health care transition: Destinations unknown. *Pediatrics, 110,* S1307-S1314.

Reiss, J. G., Gibson, R. W., & Walker, L. R. (2005). Health care transition: youth, family, and provider perspectives. *Pediatrics, 115*(1), 112-120.

Sawicki, G. S., Lukens-Bull, K., Yin, X., Demars, N., Huang, I. C., Livingood, W., ... & Wood, D. (2011). Measuring the transition readiness of youth with special healthcare needs: validation of the *TRAQ—Transition Readiness Assessment Questionnaire. Journal of Pediatric Psychology, 36*(2), 160-171.

Stam, H., Hartman, E. E., Deurloo, J. A., Groothoff, J., & Grootenhuis, M. A. (2006). Young adult patients with a history of pediatric disease: Impact on course of life and transition into adulthood. *Journal of Adolescent Health, 39,* 4-13.

Stewart, D. (2009). Transition to adult services for young people with disabilities: Current evidence to guide future research. *Developmental Medicine and Child Neurology, 51*(S4), 169-173. DOI:10.1111/j1469-8744.2009.03419.x

Tuchman, L., & Schwartz, M. (2013). Health outcomes associated with transition from pediatric to adult cystic fibrosis care. *Pediatrics, 132*(5), 847-853.

Tuchman, L. K., Schwartz, L. A., Sawicki, G. S., & Britto, M. T. (2010). Cystic fibrosis and the transition to adult medical care. *Pediatrics, 125*(3), 566-573.

U. S. Department of Health and Human Services (November, 2000). *Healthy People 2010.* 2nd *Ed. With Understanding and Improving Health and Objectives for Improving Health.* 2 vols. Washington, DC: U. S. Government Printing Office.

White, P. H., McManus, M. A., McAllister, J. W., & Cooley, W. C. (2012). A primary care quality improvement approach to health care transition. *Pediatric Annals, 41*(5), e1-e7. DOI: 103928/00904481-20120426-e1-7.

Wodka, E., & Barakat, L. (2007). An exploratory study of the relationship of family support and coping with adjustment: Implications for college students with a chronic illness. *Journal of Adolescence, 3,* 365-376.

Zullig, K. J., Valois, R. F., Huebner, E. S., & Drane, J. W. (2005). Adolescent health-related quality of life and perceived satisfaction with life. *Quality of Life Research, 14,* 1573-1584.

CHAPTER 10

Summary

Laura A. Nabors*

Health Education Program, School of Human Services, University of Cincinnati, 468 Dyer Hall, Mail Location 0068, Cincinnati, Ohio, OH 45221-0068, USA

Abstract: This brief chapter summarizes information from theory and research guiding the development of this book. The notion of a systems-based approach, that considers the child and his or her family members "in context" or as influenced by factors in their life settings underlies a family-centered and patient-centered approach to care, because it may allow mental health providers and members of the medical team to meet the child, parent, and other family members "where they are" in terms of coping with the child's illness and adjusting their lives to have new meanings and roles that incorporate the child's coping and resilience. The evidence or research base for provision of care that supports child functioning and positive development is growing and mental health professionals can receive excellent guidance from this literature. Utilizing information from the literature, networking with the medical team, school, and family can be key tools for the mental health provider to support the child.

Keywords: Child coping, context, family-centered care, networking, patient-centered care, resilience.

INTRODUCTION

Children are living longer and more fully as medical technology continues to advance children's adjustment to their chronic illness (Theis, 1999). This has expanded the role of mental health providers as children and their parents may benefit from the increased support and facilitation of adherence to the medical regimen that can occur when these experts become a part of the pediatric medical team. Mental health providers work in conjunction with the team to improve child and family understanding of and subsequent coping with the child's illness and the waxing and waning course of many diseases. Training in a hospital setting or

*Address correspondence to Laura A. Nabors:** Health Education Program, School of Human Services, University of Cincinnati, 468 Dyer Hall, Mail Location 0068, Cincinnati, Ohio, OH 45221-0068, USA; Tel: 513-556-5537; Fax: 513-556-3898; E-mail: naborsla@ucmail.uc.edu

working with children with special health care needs in community settings is recommended for those mental health providers wishing to provide specialized care in this area. Another area for specialized training is learning about interventions to help children and their family members deal with grief and loss as they must adjust to the "loss" of a normal childhood for the child who has the chronic illness. In some cases, a counselor's job is to assist the family in coping with the loss of a beloved child, and this calls for expertise in grief and loss interventions (Worden, 2009).

KEY AREAS REVIEWED IN THIS BOOK

For this text, a systems or systemic approach to understanding the child, as a member of his or her family, school, hospital, and neighborhood environments has been proposed (Bradley-Klug *et al.*, 2013; Power *et al.*, 2003). The child is reciprocally influenced by members of the medical team, school, peers, parents, and other family members. Understanding the interplay between the complex factors that determine a child's coping and reactions can facilitate understanding of ways to assist the child so that the best evidence-based interventions can be employed to foster resilience in the child. Resilience factors, such as hope and support, may also play a critical role in improving parent and family adjustment to the stress of coping with a chronic illness (McCubbin *et al.*, 2000).

Rolland (1984) wrote of having a developmental context, which considered the child, and his or her development, and the family developmental trajectory, within a systems approach to treating the child. This means that in addition to consideration of the physical contexts, the clinician should also focus on the developmental level of the child and the family as a unit. For example, "young" families, with the oldest child being ill, may react very differently than relatively "older" families, where the youngest of several children is facing a chronic illness. The older family may have developed more coping skills and have more support from siblings and enhanced financial resources to care for the child, thereby reducing their stress and improving their resilience. The notion of considering developmental stage is consistent with and at the same time broadens the reach and impact of taking a systems approach.

The role(s) of the mental health provider, who is alternately called a therapist, clinician, or counselor, are multi-faceted. The aforementioned terms may be used interchangeably if one takes a broad spectrum approach to viewing the field of mental health. However, as mentioned throughout this book, immersion in the literature and training with children and families experiencing and coping with chronic illness may be considered appropriate pre-requisites for enhancing knowledge about medical conditions and training for a position to work with children and families in hospital and community settings. There may be relatively more roles in the hospital settings, but social workers, counselors, pediatric therapists, psychologists and other mental health providers may expand their role when assisting the child and family, where they are most, which are settings within their respective day-to-day lives or communities. To place the role of pediatric therapist strictly in the hospital and not consider his or her role as a guide in various community settings may be short-changing the impact that a counselor can have in facilitating resilience and helping the family plan to deal with the child's development in his or her real-world settings.

Helping parents, siblings, extended family, and the child find new family roles and meaning in their developing lives, as they move on and function around and beyond the child's illness is another key role for the mental health professional or provider. He or she should endeavor to receive training and ongoing continuing education in grief and loss interventions. Moreover, improving knowledge in positive psychological techniques may be another way to foster resilience in the child and his or her family (Seligman & Csikszentmihalyi, 2000). Interacting with teachers, school staff, coaches, and other children in the child's class can be a way to educate those "in contact" with the child and help them find ways to incorporate the child in ongoing activities. Then, he or she can be inconspicuously a "member of the group" while still being able to care for any special needs related to his or her chronic illness or related medical regimen.

Chapters in this text addressed child coping, assessment of child functioning, parent coping, sibling coping, and the transition to adult care as other areas where mental health professionals can facilitate growth and adaptation for the child and significant others in the child's life. In terms of parent coping, assessment of parent depression and anxiety may be critical as well as being able to gain information about family support and financial situation. Honing skills for assessing parent and family functioning and coping with a chronic illness are essential abilities (Palermo & Eccleston, 2009). Supporting parents and teaching them about their child's illness, supports the child as there is a dynamic interplay among parent and child reactions to illness (Peterson & Palermo, 2004).

Many siblings cope well and have increased compassion and empathy as they assist their brother or sister. However, some can experience isolation and needs for adult attention, if they feel a parent is not spending time with them (Herzer *et al.*, 2010; Neilsen *et al.*, 2012). Assessment of factors to promote sibling resilience and finding support for the sibling through groups or at school are alternative sources for bolstering sibling adaptation should ties with parents be temporarily weakened, as the parent copes with grief and loss.

As a young adult, there is a key transition, as the patient moves to the adult care system. Close ties with the pediatric medical team need to be considered and teaching the young adult skills to explain his or her illness and advocate for his or her development are important to resilient functioning and adjustment in young adulthood. Ensuring that a portable medical summary accompanies the young adult and opening lines of communication between the pediatric and adult teams can ensure education and support of the adult care team (Stewart, 2009; Tuchman & Schwartz, 2013). Some recommend transition clinics, as a first stop in moving the young adult into the adult insurance and medical care system (Crowley *et al.*, 2011; White *et al.*, 2012).

CONCLUSION

As evidenced by the vast literature touched upon in this book there are many resources for the mental health provider. Contributing to the literature through publishing and presenting work on case studies and other clinical experiences will add to our knowledge about best practices in the care of youth with chronic illnesses. Conducting evaluations of interventions will further build the knowledge base, with a long-term goal of contributing to the literature by conducting clinical trials to determine the effectiveness of interventions to improve coping and enhance support of the child with the illness and his or her family.

ACKNOWLEDGEMENTS

None declared.

CONFLICT OF INTEREST

The author confirms that this chapter contents have no conflict of interest.

REFERENCES

Bradley-Klug, K. L., Jeffries-DeLoatche, K. L., St. John Walsh, A., Bateman, L. P., Nadeau, J., Powers, D. J., & Cunningham, J. (2013). School psychologists' perceptions of primary care partnerships: Implications for building the collaborative bridge. *Special Issue in Advances in School Mental Health Promotion, entitled, Effectively Supporting youth with chronic illness in schools, 6*(1), 51-67.

Crowley, R., Wolfe, I., Lock, K., & McKee, M. (2011). Improving the transition between paediatric and adult healthcare: A systematic review. *Archives of Disease in Childhood, 96*(6), 548-553.

Herzer, M., Godiwala, N., Hommel, K. A., Driscoll, K., Mitchell, M., Crosby, L., Piazza-Wagoner, C., Zeller, M. H., & Modi, A. C. (2010). Family functioning in the context of pediatric chronic conditions. *Journal of Developmental and Behavioral Pediatrics, 31*(1), 26-34.

McCubbin, H., Thompson, A., Futrell, J., & McCubbin, L. (Eds.). (2000). *Promoting resiliency in families and children at risk: Interdisciplinary perspectives.* Thousand Oaks, CA: Sage Publications.

Neilson, K. M., Mandleco, B., Roper, S. O., Cox, A., Dyches, T., & Marshall, E. S. (2012). Parental perceptions of sibling relationships in families rearing a child with a chronic condition. *Journal of Pediatric Nursing, 27*, 34-43.

Palermo, T. M., & Eccleston, C. (2009). Parents of children and adolescents with chronic pain. *Pain, 146*(1-2), 15-17.

Peterson, C. C., & Palermo, T. M. (2004). Parental reinforcement of recurrent pain: The moderating impact of child depression and anxiety on functional disability. *Journal of Pediatric Psychology, 29*(5), 331-341.

Power, T. J., DuPaul, G. J., Shapiro, E. S., & Kazak, A. E. (2003). *Promoting children's health: Integrating school, family, and community.* New York: Guilford Press.

Rolland, J. S. (1984). Toward a psychosocial typology of chronic life-threatening illness. *Family Systems Medicine, 2*(3), 245-262.

Seligman, M. E. P., & Csikszentmihalyi, M. (2000). Positive psychology: An introduction. *American Psychologist, 55*(1), 5-14.

Stewart, D. (2009). Transition to adult services for young people with disabilities: Current evidence to guide future research. *Developmental Medicine and Child Neurology, 51*(S4), 169-173. DOI:10.1111/j1469-8744.2009.03419.x

Thies, K. M. (1999). Identifying the educational implications of chronic illness in school children. *Journal of School Health, 69*(10), 392-397.

Tuchman, L., & Schwartz, M. (2013). Health outcomes associated with transition from pediatric to adult cystic fibrosis care. *Pediatrics, 132*(5), 847-853.

White, P. H., McManus, M. A., McAllister, J. W., & Cooley, W. C. (2012). A primary care quality improvement approach to health care transition. *Pediatric Annals, 41*(5), e1-e7. DOI: 103928/00904481-20120426-e1-7.

Worden, J. W. (2009). *Grief counseling and grief therapy: A handbook for the mental health practitioner, Fourth Edition*. New York: Springer Publishing.

INDEX

A

G

P

U

www.ingramcontent.com/pod-product-compliance
Lightning Source LLC
Chambersburg PA
CBHW041701210326
41598CB00007B/490